PICKLEBALL FUNDAMENTALS

SECOND EDITION

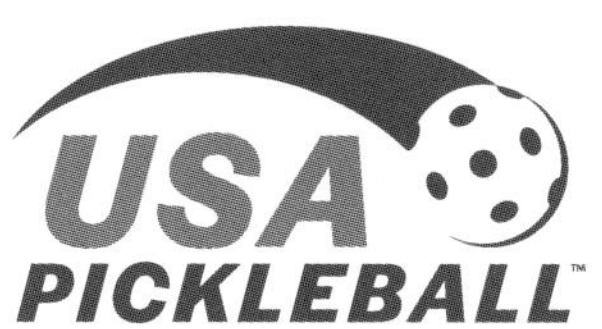

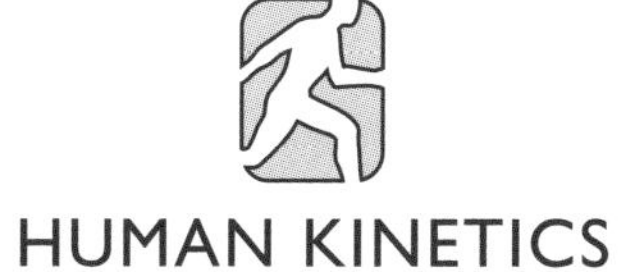

HUMAN KINETICS

Library of Congress Cataloging-in-Publication Data

Names: USA Pickleball, author.
Title: Pickleball fundamentals / USA Pickleball.
Description: Second edition. | Champaign, IL : Human Kinetics, [2025] | First edition published in 2015.
Identifiers: LCCN 2023058822 (print) | LCCN 2023058823 (ebook) | ISBN 9781718222205 (print : alk. paper) | ISBN 9781718222212 (epub) | ISBN 9781718222229 (pdf)
Subjects: LCSH: Pickleball (Game)--Handbooks, manuals, etc. | BISAC: SPORTS & RECREATION / Racket Sports / General | SPORTS & RECREATION / General
Classification: LCC GV990 .L58 2025 (print) | LCC GV990 (ebook) | DDC 796.34/8--dc23/eng/20231227
LC record available at https://lccn.loc.gov/2023058822
LC ebook record available at https://lccn.loc.gov/2023058823

ISBN: 978-1-7182-2220-5 (print)

The web addresses cited in this text were current as of December 2023, unless otherwise noted.

Acquisitions Editor: Diana Vincer; **Managing Editor:** Kevin Matz; **Project Writer:** Keith Howell; **Editorial Assistant:** Ian C. Fricker; **Copyeditor:** Laura Magzis; **Permissions Manager:** Laurel Mitchell; **Graphic Designer:** Dawn Sills; **Cover Designer:** Keri Evans; **Cover Design Specialist:** Susan Rothermel Allen; **Photograph (cover):** USA Pickleball; **Photographs (interior):** © Human Kinetics, unless otherwise noted; **Photo Production Specialist:** Amy M. Rose; **Photo Production Manager:** Jason Allen; **Senior Art Manager:** Kelly Hendren; **Illustrations:** © Human Kinetics; **Printer:** Versa Press

We thank Pictona at Holly Hill in Holly Hill, Florida, for assistance in providing the location for the photo shoot for this book.

Human Kinetics books are available at special discounts for bulk purchase. Special editions or book excerpts can also be created to specification. For details, contact the Special Sales Manager at Human Kinetics.

Printed in the United States of America 10 9 8 7 6 5 4 3 2 1

The paper in this book is certified under a sustainable forestry program.

Human Kinetics
1607 N. Market Street
Champaign, IL 61820
USA

United States and International
Website: **US.HumanKinetics.com**
Email: info@hkusa.com
Phone: 1-800-747-4457

Canada
Website: **Canada.HumanKinetics.com**
Email: info@hkcanada.com

E9170

CONTENTS

INTRODUCTION

If you are not already involved in the sport of pickleball, you're probably wondering what it is. It is an easy-to-learn game that can be played either indoors or outdoors on a badminton-size court. A seamless, perforated plastic ball the approximate size of a baseball, much like a Wiffle ball, is hit with a solid, stringless paddle—somewhat bigger than a table tennis paddle and without the rubber surface—either after one bounce or in the air. The object of the game is to hit the ball over the net, which is approximately 3 feet (about 1 m) high, to the opponent in such a way that it cannot be returned successfully. While singles (one player on each side of the net) and doubles (teams of two partners on each side) are both played, doubles is currently much more popular.

Because of its popularity, pickleball doubles play is the focus of this book, rather than singles play. Similarly, because most people are right-handed, instructions and photos are based on play by right-handed players; the assumption is that left-handed players will reverse the instructions.

Pickleball, enjoyed by players of all ages and skill levels, is soaring in popularity. More and more courts are springing up in backyards and public parks, and the game is now being taught in many schools. Colleges are forming teams and hosting interscholastic tournaments. Wealthy investors and others have seen this trend, investing money and time in everything from professional leagues, team exhibitions, and new facilities offering food, drink, and pickleball in various creative combinations, to paddle technologies, research, and improvements. This book provides you with information about the basic skills and strategies of pickleball, so that you, too, can enjoy this exciting game.

History

The game was created in 1965 by Joel Pritchard, a congressman from the state of Washington, and Bill Bell, a successful businessman, at Pritchard's home on Bainbridge Island, as a means of entertaining their respective families—in particular, their kids—during a family barbecue. An old outdoor badminton court on the property provided a place to

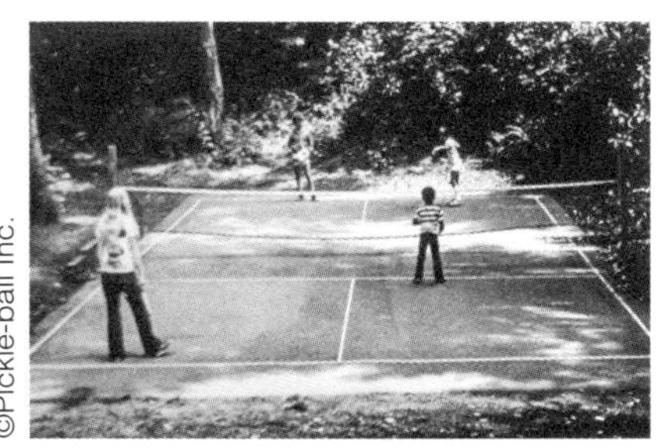
©Pickle-ball Inc.

The first pickleball court, on the Pritchards' property.

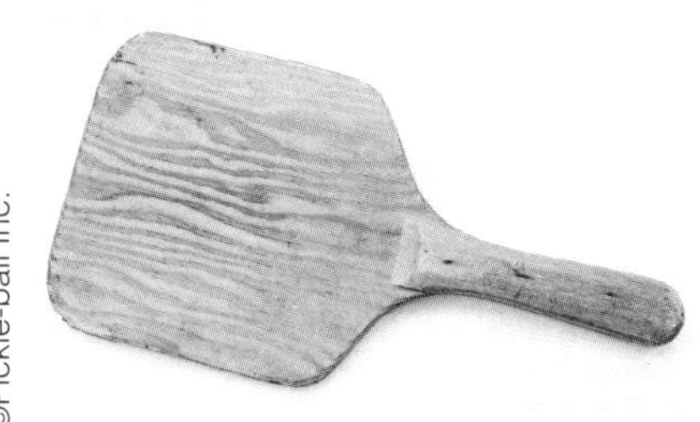
©Pickle-ball Inc.

The first wooden paddle used.

play. Family members used table tennis paddles to volley a plastic ball (unearthed during a search through rusty tools on the property) over an improvised net that was 60 inches (152 cm) high. The players soon discovered that the ball bounced nicely on the asphalt, so they lowered the net to 36 inches (91 cm). Barney McCallum was introduced to the game the following weekend while visiting the Pritchards. Pritchard, Bell, and McCallum created simple rules, staying true to the original goal of creating a game that the whole family could play together. The game they devised proved to be so much fun for the whole family that it soon became a regular weekend activity at the Pritchards'.

Accounts vary of how the name "pickleball" originated. A July 16, 2013, article in the *Wall Street Journal* says this:

> "The name comes not from the family dog, Pickles, as popularly related. According to a newspaper column by Pritchard's wife, Joan, it was so heavily based on other games it reminded her of the pickle boat in crew, "where oarsmen were chosen from the leftovers of other boats."

Popular belief as related over the years is that the game was named after the family's dog, Pickles, who chased after the ball. Others claim both accounts may actually be true. Regardless of where it came from, the name pickleball has endured.

The game gradually caught on, and the first known pickleball tournament in the world was held in spring 1976 at the South Center Athletic Club in Tukwila, Washington. Many of the participants were collegiate tennis players who knew very little about pickleball. In fact, they had practiced with large wooden paddles and a baseball-size Wiffle ball.

As more people played the game, they liked it and wanted to continue playing. The need for consistent rules, established tournament formats, and equipment standards became more important. Consequently, the USA Pickleball Association was organized in 1984, and it published the first rule book in March of that year. Now known as the USAP, it continues to serve as the national governing body of the sport. Detailed information about all aspects of pickleball, including the current rules, is available on its website, www.usapickleball.org. The International Federation of Pickleball (IFP) was formed for the purpose of standardizing pickleball competition and rules worldwide and produced its first rulebook in 2010. The USAP now recognizes the IFP's *Official Tournament Rulebook* as the official reference for competition throughout the world. It is generally updated each January 1.

In 2003, Pickleball was included for the first time in the Huntsman World Senior Games, held in St. George, Utah. The games, whose mission is to foster global peace, health, and friendship, originated in 1987. It is the largest annual multisport event in the world for athletes age 50 and older. The visibility of pickleball on that stage spurred a rise in the popularity of the sport worldwide. According to the USAP, by February 2015, pickleball was being played in all 50 U.S. states at more than 3,000 sites. It is now widely recognized as the fastest-growing sport in the world.

Court

A pickleball court is 44 feet long and 20 feet wide (13.4 by 6.1 m), the same size as a doubles badminton court. To put this into perspective, a tennis court is 78 feet (23.7 m) long and, for doubles, 36 feet (11 m) wide. Two to four pickleball courts will fit on one tennis court.

A line going from sideline to sideline on a pickleball court, 7 feet (2.1 m) from the net, designates an area called the non-volley zone (NVZ), commonly referred to by players as "the kitchen." The non-volley zone

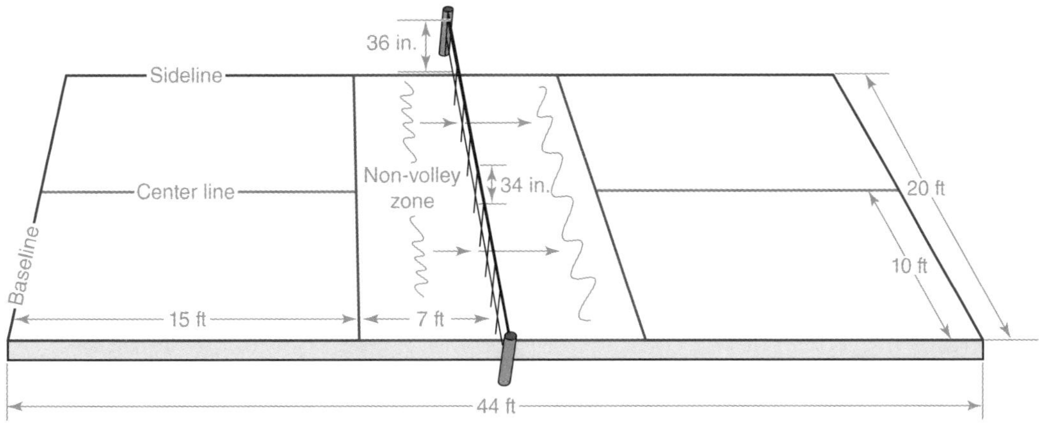

Diagram of a pickleball court.

line is considered part of the NVZ, so all rules that pertain to the NVZ apply to the line. Therefore, since a serve (the opening shot of each rally) cannot bounce anywhere in the NVZ, a served ball landing on the NVZ line is a fault. Each of the two service courts (the areas where a legal serve must land) is 15 feet long and 10 feet wide (4.6 by 3 m). The net is 36 inches high (91 cm) over the sidelines and 34 inches high (86 cm) in the center of the court.

Equipment

Very little equipment is needed for a game of pickleball. Durable paddles are available in a variety of materials and price ranges. Several brands of balls are acceptable for competition. Some are more durable than others. Standards for apparel and shoes are generally laxer in pickleball than in tennis. An overview of each category of equipment follows.

Paddles

Years ago the only choice of a pickleball paddle would have been wood, but now there are many choices. Wood paddles still exist and are sold; they are heavy, difficult to control, and not approved for tournament play. Most players prefer to use a lighter-weight paddle made of newer materials such as composite, graphite, aluminum, carbon fiber, fiberglass, or vinyl, usually sandwiched around a durable, honeycombed poly core. Paddles made of newer materials range in weight from 6 to 12 ounces (170–340 g).

Paddles also have various grip lengths and range in circumference from 4 to 4.5 inches. As a new player, you should use a paddle that is light enough for you to swing without putting undue stress on your elbow and one with a grip that is the right size for your hand. Most adult beginners would do well to start with a paddle that is 7-8.5 ounces. If you decide you later want to make an inexpensive change, special lead tape is available that adds weight to a paddle, and overgrips can add to the circumference of the grip.

Most pickleball clubs have demonstration paddles that you can use briefly if you're a new player so that you can make an intelligent choice. If that opportunity doesn't exist, some online retail companies allow a trial period of up to 30 days before you commit to the sale. And pickleball is a social sport, so many players are happy to let a newcomer try one of their own paddles.

Balls

A pickleball is made of durable, smooth, molded plastic. It is 2.75 to 3 inches (7-7.6 cm) in diameter and weighs between 0.8 and 1.02 ounces (22.7-29 g). The spacing of the holes and overall design of the ball must conform to the straight-flight and bounce characteristics required for play. Some balls are specified as being better for indoor play. Most brands of balls come in various colors as well as arrangements and sizes of holes and are available through online pickleball stores. The preferred brand of ball is determined by the tournament director, the players on the court, or the club.

Clothing and Shoes

Rules are flexible on clothing for pickleball. Any clothing that permits free movement is acceptable, as long as it is not distracting in any way and is in good taste. Shoes must have soles that do not mark or damage the playing surface.

Tennis-specific or pickleball court shoes are highly recommended. They have a nonlugged, grooved sole intended for paved or hard surfaces and are designed to provide proper support that allows a player to start, stop, and move quickly in any direction. *Running and most other types of shoes are not designed to move in this way and can lead to tripping, falling, and injury.*

Scoring and Action

Generally, the first team or player to score 11 points wins the game. That team or player must be at least 2 points ahead of the opponent. Either the player serving or the referee (if there is a referee) announces the score. A tournament match may consist of best 2 out of 3 games to 11, or one game to 15 or 21. Before the match, a coin flip, a twirl of the paddle, or some other objective means determines which team or player will serve first and on which side of the net each team will begin the match. In a 3-game match, teams switch sides at the end of the first game and, if the match should go to 3 games, when one team reaches 6 points. While these are the most accepted standards, in casual play players may adopt different scoring formats, as do some tournaments.

Doubles Scoring

In a doubles match, the player positioned behind the right-side service court of the team serving to begin a game will serve the ball. That player will continue serving from behind alternate service courts until their team commits a fault (such as a ball hit into the net). The serve will then go to the opposing team, and the player behind their right service court serves first. If their team scores a point, she serves next from behind the left service court, and that process continues until their team commits a fault. At that time, their partner serves from behind whichever service court they are positioned, based on switching sides during previous rallies. From then until the end of the game, both partners have the opportunity to serve each service turn.

The score consists of three numbers: the server's score, the serve receiving team's score, and whether it's the first or second server. The score, which should be announced before the serve to start each game, is 0-0-2. The serving team's score is 0, the serve receiving team's score is 0, and the "second" server is serving (the initial serving team gets only one fault before they lose the serve. If the serving team loses the rally, the serve goes to the opponents. From then until the end of the game, both partners have the opportunity to serve, one serving until their team faults, followed by the second partner having their turn until their team makes a second fault. The third number in the score will always be either 1 (first server of the team is serving) or 2 (second server serving). While it may seem confusing at first, after you've played a few times it will become automatic. If at least one of the four people playing on the court knows how to keep score, that's usually enough.

Singles Scoring

In a singles match, the score consists of only two numbers. The score at the start is 0-0. The player serving first serves from behind the right service court. If the server wins the rally, the score is 1-0. The serving

Rally #	Score (Serving team-Receiving team-Server)	Server (circled)	Rally winner	Results
1	0-0-2	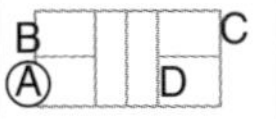 B (A) / C D	A and B	Point
2	1-0-2	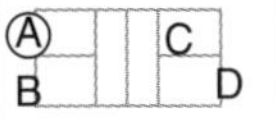 (A) B / C D	A and B	Point
3	2-0-2	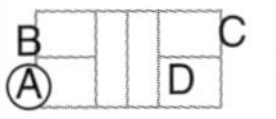 B (A) / C D	C and D	Sideout (Serve goes to opponents)
4	0-2-1	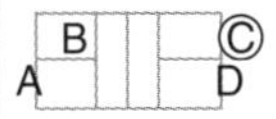 B A / (C) D	A and B	Second server
5	0-2-2	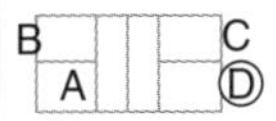 B A / C (D)	C and D	Point
6	1-2-2	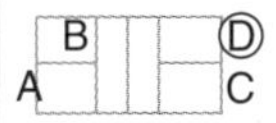 B A / (D) C	A and B	Sideout
7	2-1-1	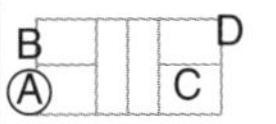 B (A) / D C	A and B	Point
8	3-1-1	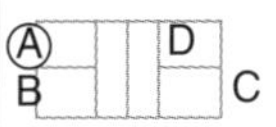 (A) B / D C	C and D	Second server
9	3-1-2	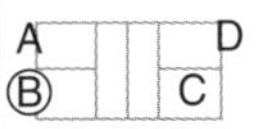 A (B) / D C	A and B	Point

Doubles scoring chart.

player's score is always given first. The server then serves from behind the left service court. If that player continues to win rallies, they continue serving from behind alternate service courts. If they lose the rally, the serve goes to the opponent, who serves from behind the court that is determined by the score. When a player's score is even, the serve is from behind the right service court; when their score is odd, the serve is from behind the left service court.

Etiquette

Many of the rules of etiquette and good conduct for pickleball are common to all sports. Most important is to remember your objective in playing the game. While it is widely written that playing should be fun, you know that it's more fun if you play up to your capabilities. Doing your best is all that should be expected of you. Being able to accept graciously a loss as well as a win is the true gauge of good sporting behavior.

- Be on time for matches.
- If you are playing on a court that requires you to walk through another court that is in use, be sure that their play is stopped before you enter their court.
- Agree with your opponents about the warm-up procedure you'll follow before a match.
- Make all line calls on your side of the net fairly, giving your opponents the benefit of the doubt on close calls. The ball should be clearly out before it is called as out. If partners disagree about whether the ball is in or out, it is deemed in, and the rally should go to the opponents.
- The player with the best position and angle should make the line call. Ideally, you should watch the lines for balls going toward your partner so they can concentrate fully on their shot. Remember, one line call, whether good or bad, does not win or lose a game.
- Many locations have traditions and local "house rules." These may involve who plays next with whom, which side serves first, what happens if the ball hits an overhanging object, or whether one should catch an "out" ball before it bounces to prevent it hindering play on an adjacent court. As a newcomer, it's a good idea to ask for guidance from a local, more experienced player. It usually can be as simple as, "Hi. It's my first time here. How do I get in a game?"

A Word About the Book's Structure

This book contains information, instructions, photos, and illustrations that will help you immerse yourself in the sport of pickleball. The bulk of the information is in four sections:

- *You can do it*: Get a clear explanation of how to perform an essential skill or tactic.
- *More to choose and use*: Find out more and explore alternatives.
- *Take it to the court*: Apply the new skill in a hands-on situation.
- *Give it a go*: Use a drill or activity to hone or expand the fundamental techniques outlined in the chapter.

The key on page xvii explains the player designations in the illustrations.

Apply the techniques and tactics as you learn them, and have fun!

KEY TO DIAGRAMS

D	Player executing a dink
DS	Player executing a drop shot
DV	Player executing a drop volley
HV	Player executing a half volley
F	Feeder
L	Player executing a lob
OS	Player executing an overhead smash
P	Any player
PA	Player A in a doubles match or drill
PB	Player B in a doubles match or drill
PC	Player C in a doubles match or drill
PD	Player D in a doubles match or drill
R1	Receiver
R2	Receiver's partner
S1	Server
S2	Server's partner
SP	Stronger player on a doubles team
(T)	Target
V	Player executing a volley
WP	Weaker player on a doubles team
	Balls
——➤	Path of player
- - -➤	Initial path of ball
- - -➤	Secondary path of ball
- - -➤	Path of ball
●	Bounce (small solid circle)
	Ball hopper

CHAPTER

1

Getting Ready to Play (and Staying That Way)

Before you participate in any sport or activity that is more strenuous than your everyday life, you need to spend at least a few minutes warming up your body—muscles, ligaments, and tendons, heart, lungs, and brain. Pickleball is no exception. Warming up with dynamic motions before playing pickleball and cooling down afterward not only helps prevent muscle soreness—a phenomenon that traditionally occurs a day or so after exertion—but can also help to prevent injuries. If, like many busy teens and adults, you do not participate in regular exercise, you may find that your muscles, joints, and connective tissues are less pliable and require more conditioning. This makes taking care of your body before and after pickleball even more important.

Focused stretching exercises, particularly the static "reach and hold the position for a count of 10" versions, have been a mainstay of physical education for decades, but research is now showing their limits. Many experts are now recommending that this kind of stretching be done after a workout is complete (if at all), when the body is fully warmed up. While it is always wise to consult with a reputable professional for specific recommendations directed at your individual physical health and age, we will discuss here some basic dynamic warm-up exercises that will benefit any pickleball player.

You Can Do It

WARMING UP

The warm-up increases circulation of the blood, which in turn carries oxygen to the cells efficiently. It gets the entire body prepared for the more vigorous movements to come. It also raises overall body temperature as well as the temperature of the deep muscles. That raised temperature allows for greater flexibility of the affected muscles and tendons, which means that they can better resist any trauma to the tissues caused by sudden extensions or unexpected motions. For this reason, always warm up thoroughly before you play.

Your body needs to be thoroughly warmed before you stretch. This means that static stretches aren't recommended as part of a warm-up. Instead, use dynamic motions that increase flexibility and add any static stretching after you are finished playing.

Warm-up activities can be of a general nature, such as walking at a quick pace or jogging, biking from home to the pickleball courts, walking on a treadmill, riding a stationary bike, or a combination of these activities. Or the warm-up activities can be more specific to the sport. Any exercise involving the upper body (particularly the arms and shoulders) as well as the lower body would be appropriate for pickleball. For instance, circling the arms from the shoulders as you walk or jog or riding a stationary bike with moving handlebars would be good warm-up exercises specific to pickleball. Be sure to warm up long enough to break a sweat or at least feel your heart pumping harder than normal and make sure you have warmed up the legs, core, and shoulders as well as any areas your own body needs. We will go over several simple but effective exercises that can get you ready to play.

More to Choose and Use

GETTING READY TO PLAY

Generally, start with whole-body exercises and ones emphasizing large muscle groups like the thighs and core before moving on to your extremities. This safely but quickly increases your heart rate, breathing, and circulation, sending extra oxygen and warmth to your entire body. Developing a regular routine ensures that every part of the body is included, so many people prefer repeating the same pattern every time they warm up. Journaling both your warm-ups and experiences during play is a great way to keep track of your progress, physically and competitively, and spot any areas you may need to work on.

Following are some suggestions for warm-up exercises. If you have injuries or particular physical conditions that make certain movements difficult, substitute motions that work for you, while making sure all the main body parts receive a thorough but gentle warm-up. The suggestions here need no equipment like rollers, bands, or weights, just your body. However, if you already have a sensible warm-up routine that works for you using these tools, do what works for you.

Do *not* "bounce" (bob up and down) or push a motion to the point that it hurts. "No Pain No Gain" does not apply to either warming up or to playing pickleball.

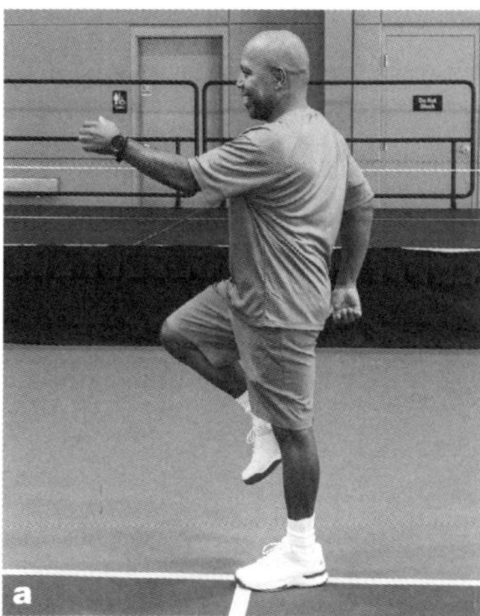

General Warm-Ups

Start with a vigorous walk, swinging your arms or circling them from your shoulders (figure 1.1*a*). An exercise bike that works the arms, an elliptical machine, or a slow jog are good substitutes. If walking, you can add marching, with knees raised to around hip or waist height as you feel your body warming (see figure 1.1*b*). Another familiar dynamic whole-body exercise that can be adjusted for differing fitness and intensity levels is the jumping jack. Do some combination of these for at least a few minutes, making sure you break a sweat or feel your respiration and heart rate increasing.

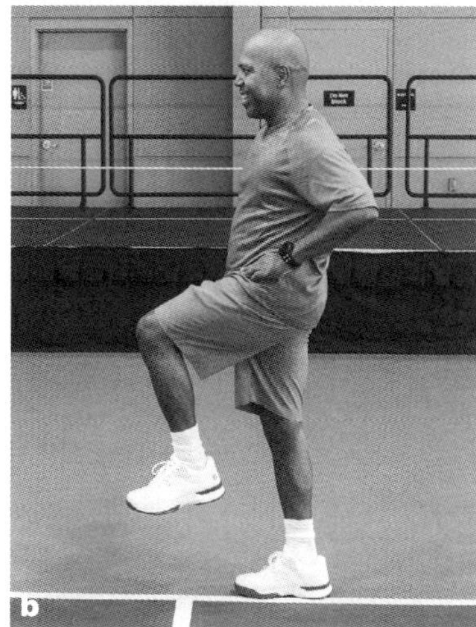

Figure 1.1 Marching, knees raised, arms swinging.

Squats

Squats are a great way to warm up and work out your lower body, hips, and core. Stand with your feet about hip width apart. Clasp your hands in front of you, out from your chest (much like the pickleball "ready" position we will be talking about later). Engage your stomach muscles while sitting down on an imaginary chair behind you, shifting your weight back onto your heels as you keep your chest out and up. Go no further down than when you feel your heels start to rise off the floor or your chest and shoulders start to round or lean forward. Your knees should not extend past your toes (figure 1.2*a-b*).

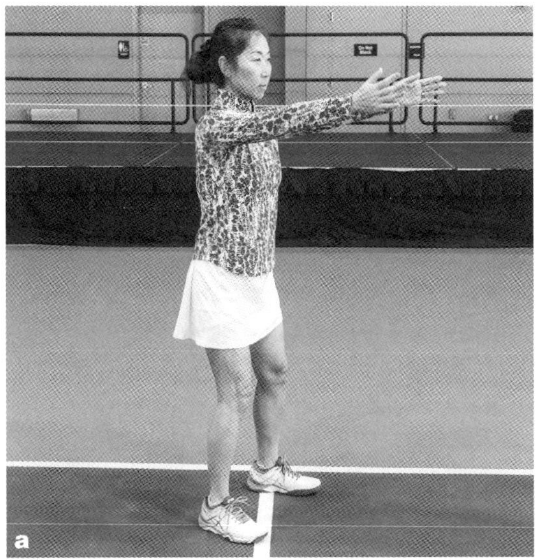

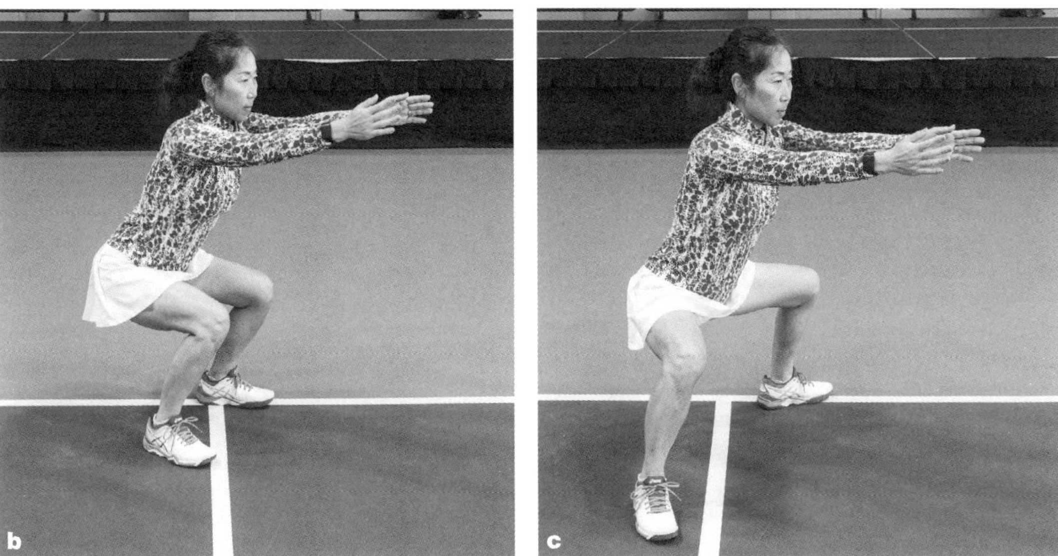

Figure 1.2 Squatting, weight back, knees staying over the feet.

Stand up in a controlled motion, keeping your chest out, shoulders square, while pushing down through your heels. Your core muscles should stay engaged the entire time. As an option, you may alternate feet, stepping out to each side about 1 foot (30 cm) for a wider-stance squat. This replicates a movement often needed to reach the ball in game play (see figure 1.2*c*). Repeat 10-15 times.

Lunges, Front-Back and Side-to-Side

Start standing, with feet about hip width apart. Step forward with one foot, striding out farther than a normal step to land with the forward foot flat on the ground, the rear foot's heel rising (figure 1.3). Lower yourself over the extended foot with control and balance, bending the front knee to about 90 degrees. Your shoulders and torso should stay upright and core tight.

Push off from your front foot with enough force to return to the standing position. Lunges can be done with the hands on top of the forward, flexing knee, clasped in front of your chest, or at your sides. Repeat 10-15 times, alternating left and right foot forward.

If it is easier at first, you can also start after the stride, with one foot staying forward, lowering your body down by flexing both knees to about 90 degrees, then pushing down into both feet to return upright. For this "'static" lunge, the feet will remain in one position for the repetitions, before you switch which foot is forward.

Just as for the squats, the knee should not extend past the foot while doing either of these lunges.

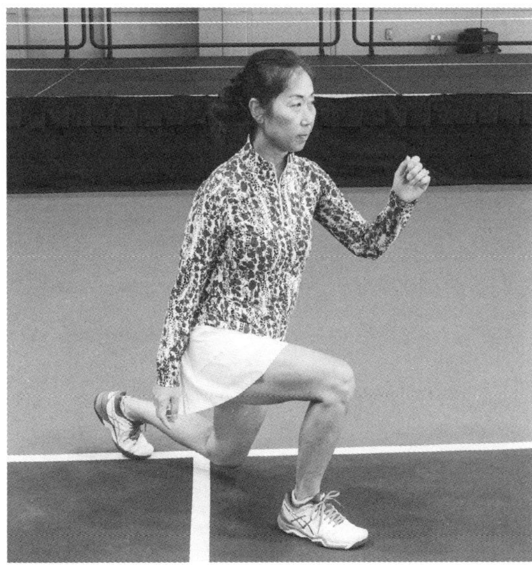

Figure 1.3 Lunge, forward.

Arm Circles

This exercise is another good way to loosen the arms and shoulders. Extend your arms to the side with the palms facing down (figure 1.4). Make small circles with the arms 8 to 10 times forward and then 8 to 10 times backward. Then repeat the exercise with larger circles reaching overhead and down near the outside of the thigh.

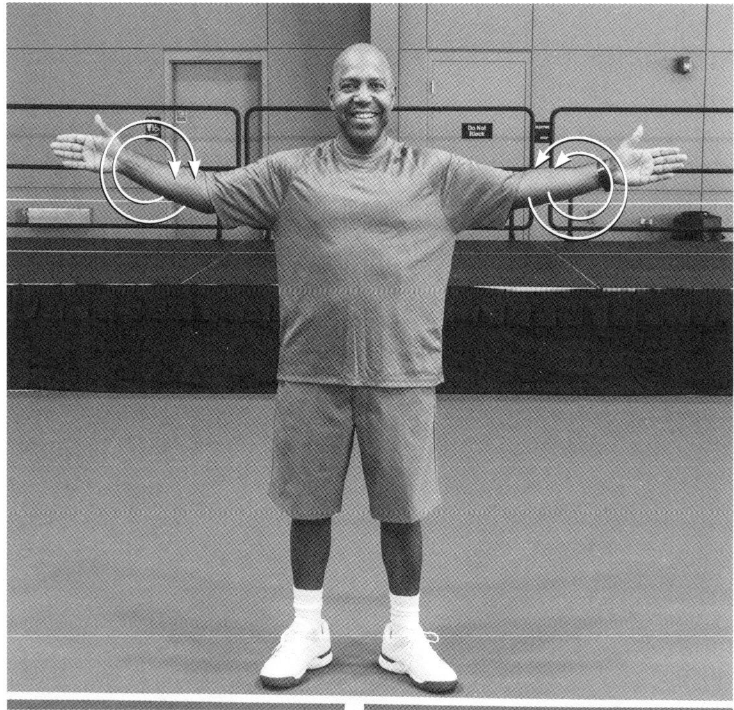

Figure 1.4 Arm circle stretch.

While most of the body positions and movements required for playing a game of pickleball are predictable, some movements require a body part to stretch farther than is comfortable. You need to warm up before beginning a game and prepare your body to handle any movements that you might face in a heated rally. A common, unexpected movement in games is reaching forward or to the side with the paddle arm while taking a sudden lunging step, almost like a fencer thrusting. This type of movement is often used as a player attempts to reach a ball that drops just over the net or almost out of their reach. Warming up the legs, hips, and shoulders well before the game will enable you to perform this action safely from the very first rally.

Take It to the Court

SAFETY PRECAUTIONS

Regardless of how conscientious you are in terms of warming up and stretching, situations will arise that could cause an injury or accident. Active, enthusiastic players who don't always communicate with one another while swinging paddles on a shared court that is only 20 feet wide can easily collide, possibly causing a variety of injuries from pulled or bruised muscles to scrapes and lacerations requiring stitches. Even though players might take every precaution to prevent a traumatic event, accidents do happen. Following are some safety precautions that if practiced will help you to prevent injury.

- *Make communicating with your partner your top priority when you play doubles.* Even if it seems obvious who should take the ball, call it out as either "Yours" or "Mine."
- *Wear eye protection, whether or not you wear glasses.* During a heated rally at the net, the ball could easily come toward your face so fast that you don't have time to get your paddle up to protect it. No part of your body is more important to protect than your eyes! While there are many brands of protective eyewear available, many players who do not need prescription glasses wear sturdy over-the-counter sunglasses or even just the frames with the lenses popped out as inexpensive eye protection.
- *Never backpedal to get to a ball.* When a shot like a soft, arcing lob lands behind you, it's too easy to trip, fall backward, and try to catch yourself with your hand. This could easily result in a head injury or a broken bone in your wrist or arm. If you have to go back to get to a ball, turn first in that direction and then run back. If you are chasing a lob, it is safer to cover a ball landing diagonally behind your partner, turning partway, rather than one directly behind yourself where you need to turn 180 degrees.
- *Listen to your body.* Pay attention to sore muscles, aching joints, and fatigue. Playing pickleball could cause further damage to whichever body part is screaming! Pain does not equal gain.
- *Never try for a ball that you can't safely get to.* It's not worth it if you lose your balance, fall, and injure yourself or someone else. Keep your feet under your body at all times and use common sense about what you're capable of.

- *Be aware of the weather conditions and dress accordingly.* Stay hydrated before and during play in hot temperatures and wear light-colored clothing that reflects the sun. Wear a hat or cap. If you will be playing in cold temperatures, dress in layers. As your body temperature varies, you can remove or add your clothing a layer at a time, contributing to a comfortable and healthy playing temperature at all times. While thinking about the weather, remember that even a slight bit of water on smooth court surfaces can be surprisingly slippery.
- *Athletic court shoes with good support, designed for quickly stopping or moving in any direction, are the safest shoes to wear on a pickleball court.* Shoes for tennis, usually called court shoes (and now many shoe brands are producing very similar pickleball shoes expressly for the sport), are usually the best choice for most players, while volleyball and basketball shoes can be another good choice if playing on wooden gym floors. Running, walking, or hiking shoes or any other type of shoe that has a deeply ridged or knobby sole can cause you to trip on the playing surface. *Running shoes are not designed or constructed to safely support the quick stopping and sideways accelerations common to pickleball.*

THE FIRST GAME OF THE DAY

It is a common tradition in pickleball to give any player playing their first recreational game of the day, or after a prolonged break, time for a brief warm-up on the court. Many players use this opportunity to chat and introduce themselves while dinking the ball idly back and forth over the net. *Use this time!* Squat deeper than usual, slow and controlled, while you return each of your dinks, using both wide and narrow stances. Work in some lunges as you reach for shots that fall short or take you out wide. Exaggerate shoulder motions, footwork, follow-throughs. Suggest hitting a few drops, drives, and serves before starting the actual game. These steps will help ensure that your entire body is ready for the action from the first rally.

Note: each of the shots and exercises mentioned above will be covered in the following pages.

Give It a Go

COOLING DOWN

As with any other athletic endeavor, allow a cool-down period after playing pickleball. Cooling down after physical activity permits both the circulation and various body functions to gradually return to preexercise levels. A few minutes' worth of any mild activity—such as gentle stretching, walking, or easy swimming or biking—will accomplish that.

You should establish a regular routine that includes a thorough dynamic warm-up before playing pickleball and a cool-down after play. Don't forget to stay moving or warm up again if you are waiting between games. Too many players take a seat to watch their friends play and forget to stay warmed up. It's easy to become so engrossed in the fun and excitement of the game itself that you become complacent about the care and attention you should give to your body before, during, and after playing.

Pickleball can be played as a casual game with little movement on the court. It can also be very intense, athletic, and competitive. Whether you are a highly competitive player who instinctively goes for every ball on your side of the court, or a casual player content to simply enjoy hitting the ball with friends, your warm-up can give your body the best possible chance of finishing that game and many more in the best possible condition.

Match Point

Spending the time and energy to warm up, cool down, and take proper precautions on and off the court as part of a pickleball playing routine is invaluable in preventing injury. Preparing your body for the physical exertion required for playing a competitive game of pickleball, cooling down gradually after you play, and following the recommended safety precautions will increase your enjoyment and extend your time on the court.

CHAPTER

2

Ready Position, Grips, and Ball Control

Key to your ability to play pickleball with any degree of success is to begin in a good ready position from which you can handle any ball that you are responsible for returning. From the ready position, you should be able to move to the ball, execute the appropriate shot using a relaxed, comfortable grip on the paddle and good ball control, and then return to a balanced position with the paddle in a ready position, prepared for the next shot. Being able to anticipate the next shot will help you judge where on the court you will need to be in order to then execute an effective return shot. Most important for success in a game is to keep the ball in play!

You Can Do It

READY POSITION

You assume the ready position (figure 2.1) in preparation for the ball coming to you from the opposite side of the net, and it is crucial to the success of your subsequent shot. When you are deep in the court (near the baseline, away from the net), you should assume a balanced, comfortable position with your feet about shoulder width apart (figure 2.1*a*). Your weight should be on the balls of your feet, and you should hold the paddle in front of your body in a relaxed but ready position. Your knees should be slightly bent and you should feel light on your feet—ready to move in any direction quickly and smoothly. Your eyes, paddle, and upper body should be tracking the ball as it crosses the net in both directions.

Your ready position when you are at the non-volley zone (NVZ) line differs slightly from the position assumed deep in your court. When you're close to the net, you should hold the paddle with a relaxed grip, extended comfortably in front of you, at about the height of your solar plexus, where your ribcage ends and the abdomen begins (figure 2.1*b*), so that it's in a good position to return hard-hit balls that just clear the net. If your paddle is too low or at your side, it takes too much time to move it into a strong volleying position, and you are likely to either

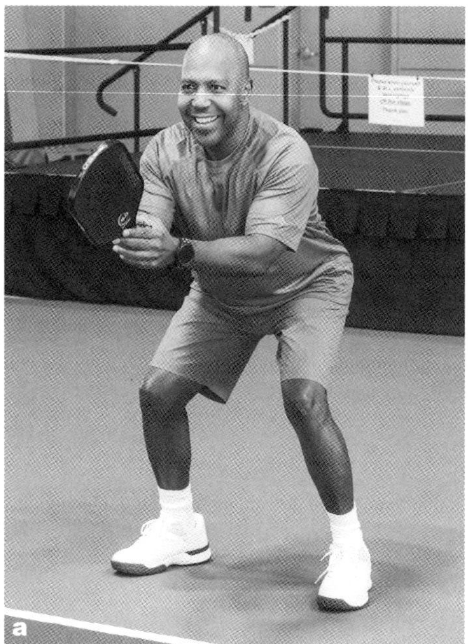

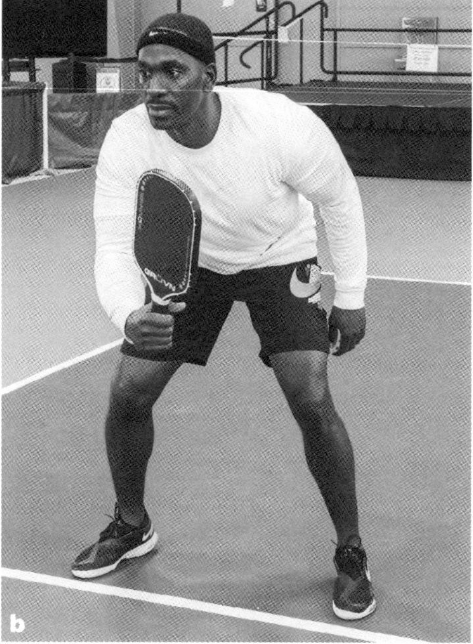

Figure 2.1 Ready position (*a*) deep in the court and (*b*) at the net.

hit an erratic shot or hit the ball into the net. The stance at the NVZ is also a little lower, with the knees bent and feet slightly wider than the shoulders.

The key to assuming a good ready position, regardless of where you are on the court, is to be balanced and ready for any shot that an opponent might hit. Always expect the ball to come to you and be ready for it! The following checklist highlights key aspects of the ready position.

Checklist for ready position.

- *Feet* are shoulder width apart or a little wider as you approach the net.
- *Knees* are slightly bent.
- *Weight* is on the balls of the feet.
- *Hands* hold the paddle in a relaxed position in front of the body when playing deep in the court.
- *Hands* hold the paddle slightly higher in front of the body when playing at the net.
- *Grip* is relaxed but secure.
- *Body* is balanced and loose—ready to move!
- *Eyes* and *paddle* are tracking the ball.

More to Choose and Use

FOREHAND GRIPS

Hold the paddle in your dominant hand with the head of the paddle perpendicular to the ground and the handle facing you. Pretend to shake hands with the paddle, curling your fingers around the rubber grip with the V formed by the thumb and the base of your index finger on top (figure 2.2). The grip should be relaxed, firm but not tight. Your dominant hand on the rubber grip should feel comfortable and in control. If this is not the case, the grip might be too small or too large for the size of your hand, and you should consider trying a paddle with a different-sized grip. If the grip is too small, you can also wrap the factory grip with an overgrip, a thin rubbery material designed to absorb sweat and make the grip less slippery. Many players find that the slight increase in the grip's size makes it easier to hold the paddle securely without straining, easing tension on the muscles and tendons of the forearm. Consider replacing your grip or overgrip occasionally as they can become worn or saturated with heavy use.

Some players extend the index finger at an angle up the back of the paddle (figure 2.3), feeling this position gives them better control of the head of the paddle and enables them to more easily apply spin on the ball. A disadvantage of a finger on the back of the paddle is that it may restrict the ability to use wrist action when contacting the ball. Many good players will shift their grip depending on what kind of shot they plan to execute, sometimes without realizing it. New players should use the standard grip while learning the game. After developing consistent skills, you can experiment with variations of the standard grip. The grip that you use is completely dependent on what is comfortable and works for you.

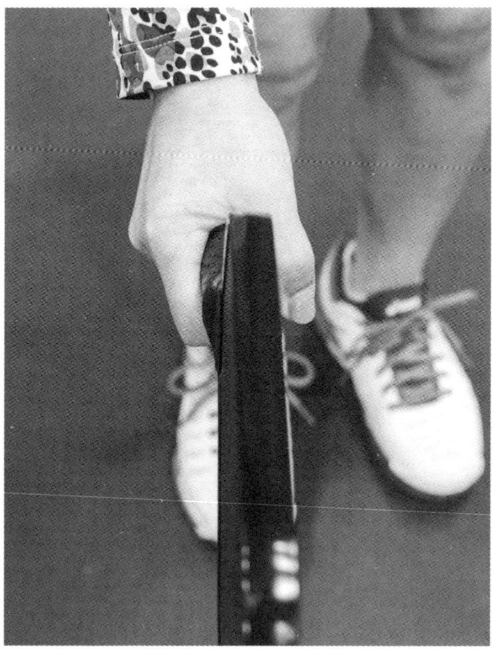

Figure 2.2 Standard forehand grip.

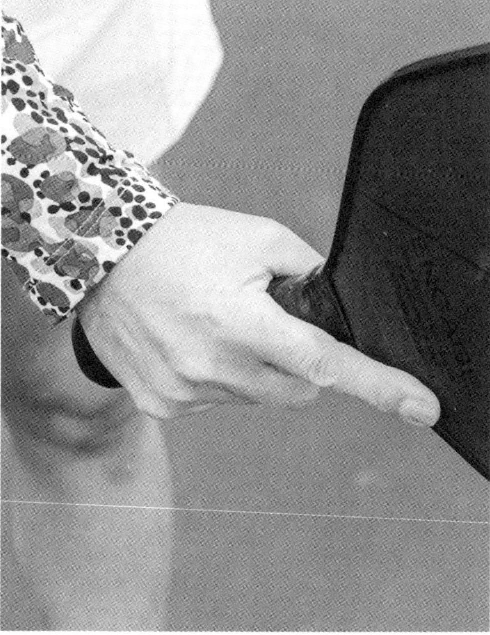

Figure 2.3 Alternative forehand grip: index finger angled up the back of the paddle.

BACKHAND GRIPS

Some players adjust the grip on the paddle for hitting a backhand shot and others do not. It is a matter of personal preference. To change the grip for a backhand shot, turn your hand slightly to the left, or counterclockwise (for a right-handed player), from a perpendicular position to the ground (figure 2.4*a*). This should occur as you're preparing for your next shot—holding the paddle in front of you in both hands with your dominant hand on the grip and the other hand above that on the neck or near the top edge of the paddle. More competitive players, especially those coming from a tennis background, are using a two-handed backhand, with the nondominant hand stabilizing the swing and allowing more topspin (figure 2.4*b*).

If you lack strength in your hands and your grip is weak, try wearing a racquetball glove on the paddle hand as an alternate to a tacky overgrip. The glove should be snug and have a tacky surface in the palm area. The tackiness of the glove helps you to grip the paddle firmly and gives you better control of the movement of the paddle.

Most important when determining the best grip is to select one that is comfortable and allows for good control of the paddle. If it works, use it!

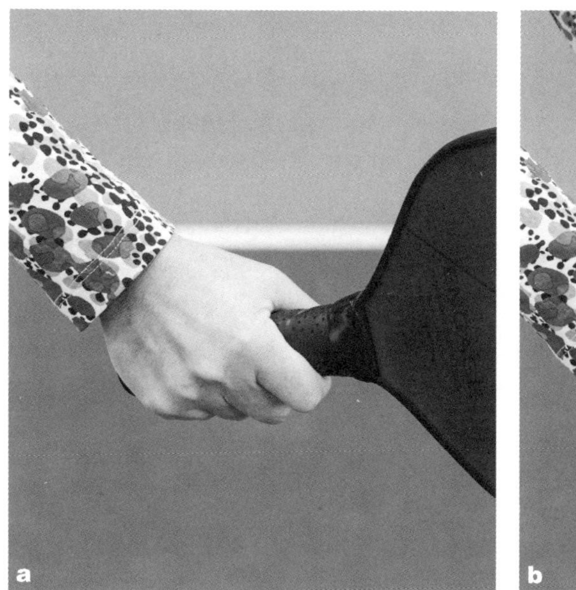

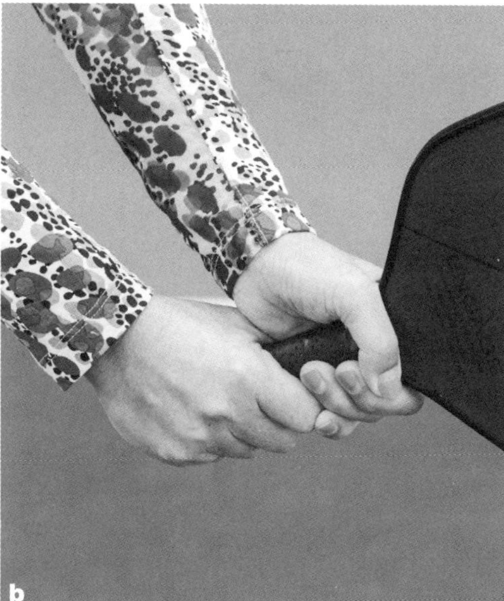

Figure 2.4 *(a)* One-handed and *(b)* two-handed backhand grips.

Take It to the Court

BALL CONTROL

In the past, many players believed there was only one correct way to play pickleball: as a game of finesse based largely on soft, controlled shots at the net (called dinks), with both doubles partners positioned just behind the NVZ line, facing the action on the other side of the net. From this position, they hit the ball softly, just over the top of the net, waiting until someone made an error by hitting it too high (an "attackable" shot), allowing their opponent to hit an aggressive, offensive shot that would be very difficult to return, thus winning the rally. While being able to hit soft dinks consistently and control the speed and direction of the ball as it comes off the face of the paddle are crucial to success in pickleball, today's game sees more aggressive, attacking play intended to force the opponents to make a mistake rather than simply waiting for the opponents to hit an attackable (too high) ball.

In the following photos, note the position of the paddle in relation to the position of the player. Although the player is always facing the net, the paddle might be square to the net in a position to contact the ball off their front knee, causing the ball to travel straight over the net (figure 2.5*a*); or, if the face of the paddle is to the right and the ball contact is opposite the right hip, the ball will travel to the right and possibly go out of bounds (2.5*b*); or the face of the paddle is to the left with the ball contact in front of the player's body, causing the ball to travel to the left (2.5*c*). Beginning players should focus on hitting their shots with the paddle squarely facing the ball, advanced players will sometimes purposely change the angle of their paddle faces to mislead their opponents.

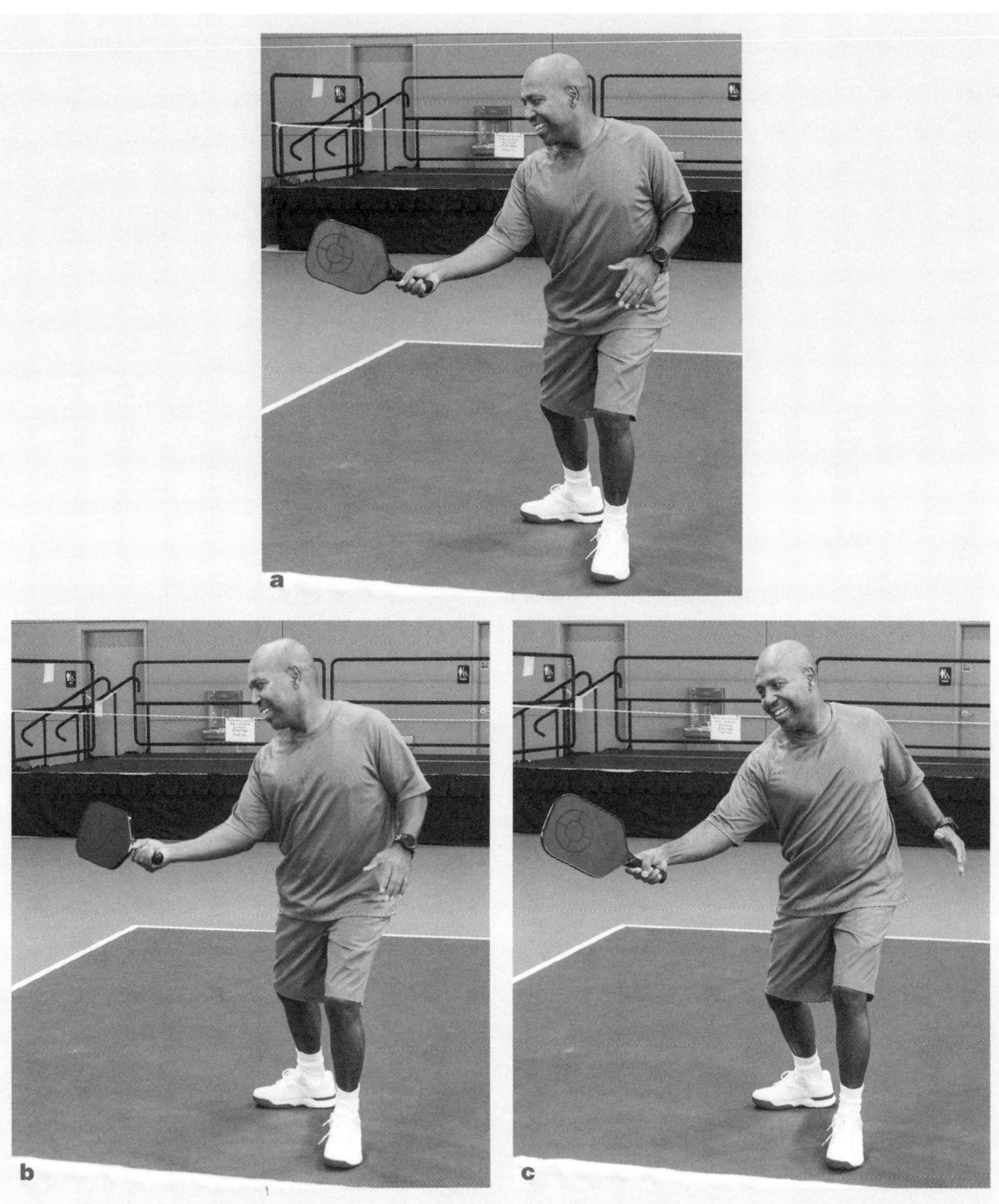

Figure 2.5 (*a*) Ball will go toward the net, (*b*) ball will go to the right, and (*c*) ball will go to the left.

Here are some principles of good ball control to learn and focus on:

- Track the ball with your eyes all the way to the face of the paddle. See it not only contact the paddle but also leave the paddle. Keep your eyes on the ball.
- Assuming that the paddle is traveling in a flat plane before contacting the ball, the ball will always leave the paddle at a 90-degree angle, perpendicular to the paddle face.
- If the arm swings upward, the ball will travel in an upward direction.
- If the arm swings downward, the ball will travel in a downward direction. If the face of the paddle is *square,* the ball will travel straight ahead, parallel to the ground (figure 2.6*a*); when the face is *open*, the ball will travel upward (2.6*b*); and when the face is *closed*, the ball will travel downward (2.6*c*).

As you execute the ball control drills, concentrate on how you move your feet to get to the ball. Since a pickleball is plastic with holes in it, it does not bounce as high or travel as far as a tennis ball or racquetball. Therefore, you have to move to the ball—the ball won't come to you. Use controlled, comfortable steps and always try to be balanced with your feet under your body when you contact the ball. The farther you are from the net when you contact the ball, the more important it is to step into the hit. Transfer your body weight from the back foot to the front foot as your paddle arm swings forward to hit the ball.

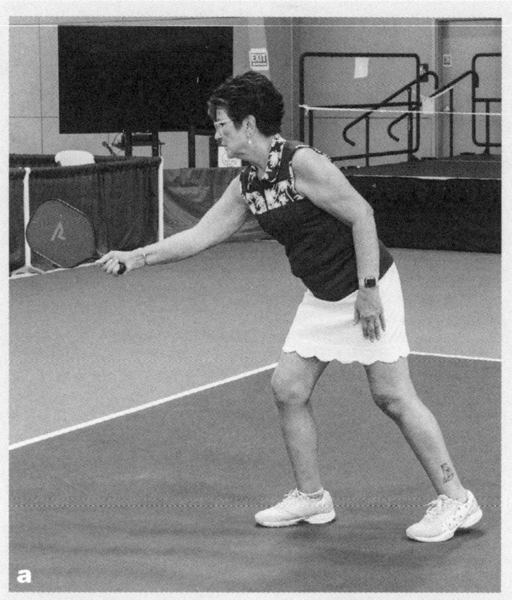

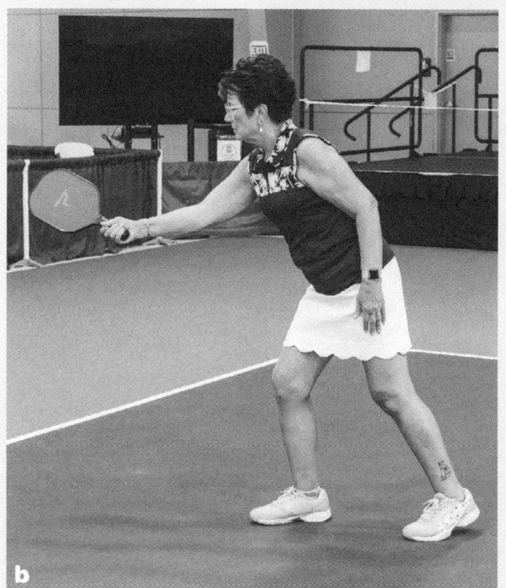

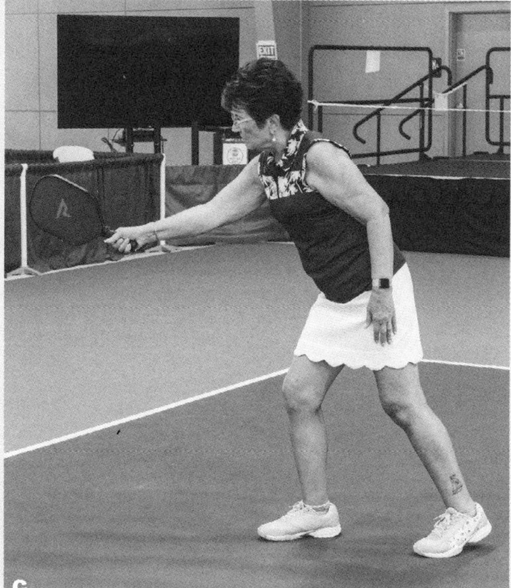

Figure 2.6 (*a*) Square, (*b*) open, and (*c*) closed paddles.

Give It a Go

Following are some drills for one player, two players, or a group of players for the purpose of practicing ball control. Emphasize throughout all of the drills that the goal is to accomplish the task, whether it's hitting a ball off the paddle, hitting to a partner, or hitting to a target. Ideally it should be a soft, controlled shot.

YO-YO UP

A single player taps the ball into the air off the paddle, trying to keep it going as long as possible. The drill is performed first with the palm of the paddle hand facing up (figure 2.7*a*), then with the palm of the paddle hand facing down (2.7*b*), and then with alternating up and down paddle positions.

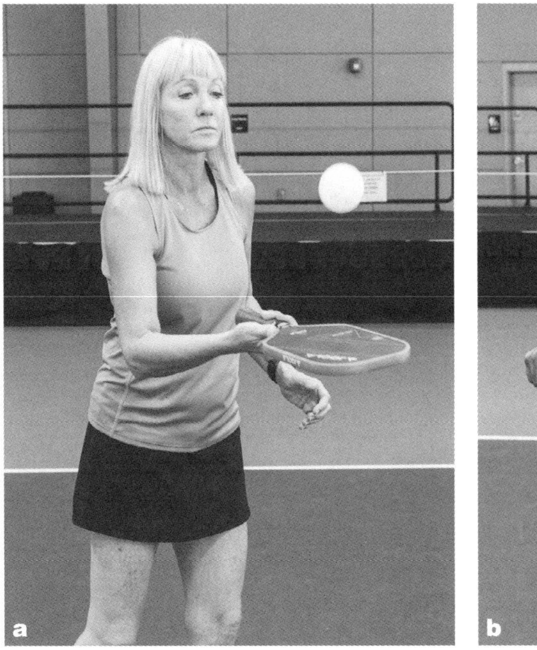

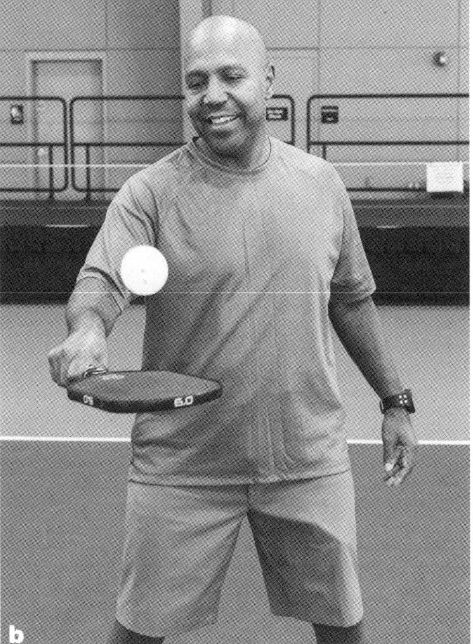

Figure 2.7 Yo-yo up drill: (*a*) palm facing up and (*b*) palm facing down.

YO-YO DOWN

A single player hits the ball to the ground, trying to execute as many consecutive bounces as possible (figure 2.8). Then alternate between one hit into the air and one hit to the ground.

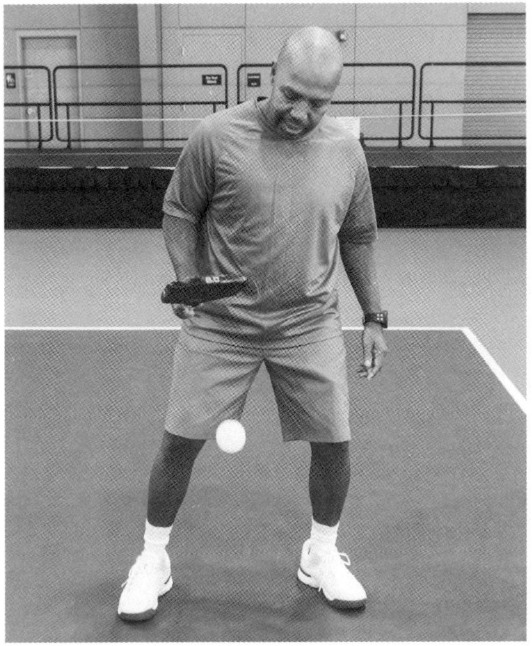

Figure 2.8 Yo-yo down drill.

HIT TO A PARTNER

Two players stand facing each other, about 8 to 10 feet apart (about 3 meters), with no net between them. The first player hits the ball, lofting it into the air; the other player hits it before it touches the ground. Players try to keep the exchange going as long as possible. Alternatively, they can try bouncing the ball to each other. If this exercise is too easy for players coming from other racket and paddle sports, it can be done over the net, either keeping the ball in the air or trying to bounce it after a short arc over the net.

PARTNERS ACROSS AND BACK

Players line up in two lines, one on each side of the court in the area of the NVZ line. A supply of balls is at the head of each line. The first players in each line (P1 and P2) move onto the court, and one player (P1), who has a ball, immediately bounces the ball and hits it to a partner on the other side of the net (figure 2.9). The two players move across the width of the court while hitting the ball back and forth. As soon as the first two players finish, they form a line on that side of the court. When all players have traveled the width of the court, they do the same thing coming back. If there are two courts available side by side, continue this drill across the two courts instead of only one.

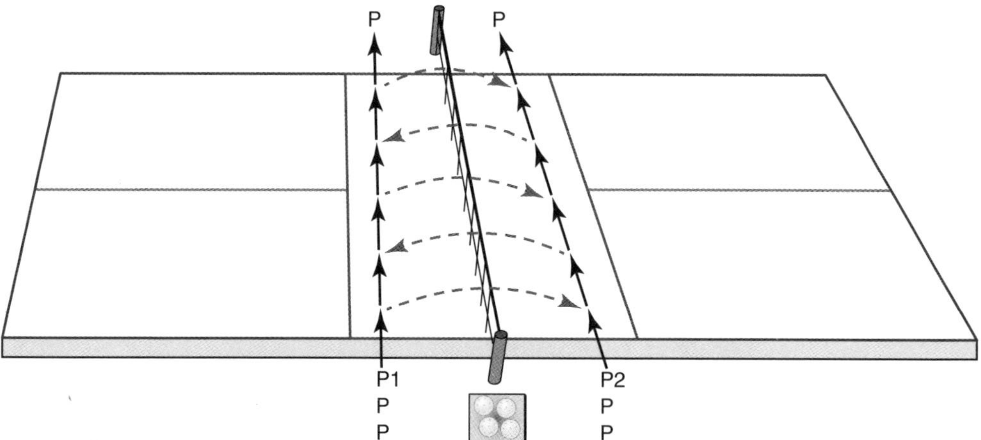

Figure 2.9 Partners across and back drill.

HIT TO A TARGET

A player (P) stands facing the net in the ready position. On the other side of the net is a feeder (F), who should be capable of throwing balls with some consistency. Targets (T) are marked on the court—these can be temporary chalk marks, towels laid flat, or movable, flat rubber targets available commercially. The target locations and target sizes should enable the participating players to be successful. The feeder tosses a ball to bounce in front of player P. That player hits the ball off the bounce, trying to hit one of the targets. On the next attempt, they should aim for the second target and then the third. The feeder should concentrate on tossing the balls consistently so the player can focus on watching the ball all the way in until it contacts the face of the paddle, then returning immediately to the ready position. The details of "proper" form are not important at this point (figure 2.10).

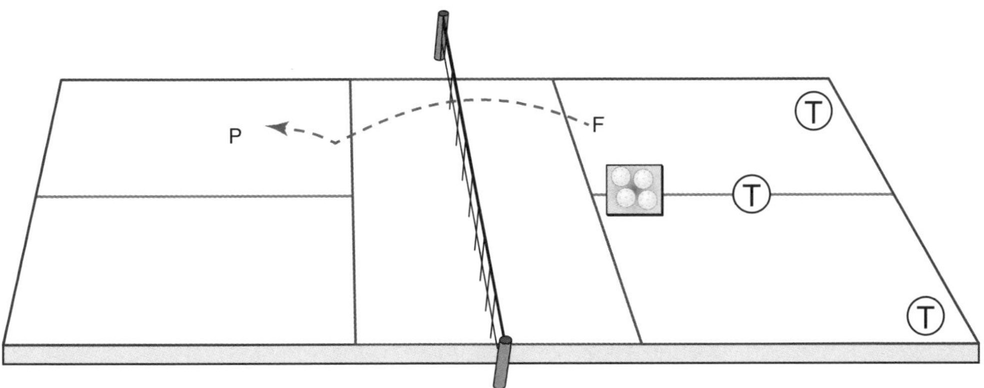

Figure 2.10 Hit to a target drill.

RALLY AT THE NET

Four players (PA, PB, PC, and PD) take the court just behind the NVZ line; players A and D set up directly across from one another, and players B and C do the same. Player A bounces the ball and hits it to player B; player B lets the ball bounce once and then hits it to player C; player C lets the ball bounce once and hits it to player D, who lets the ball bounce once and sends it back to player A (figure 2.11). Players keep the rally going as long as possible, each attempting to hit the ball in a controlled manner to the next player. The four players rotate counterclockwise, and player A starts the rally again. The rotation process continues until each player has played in each position.

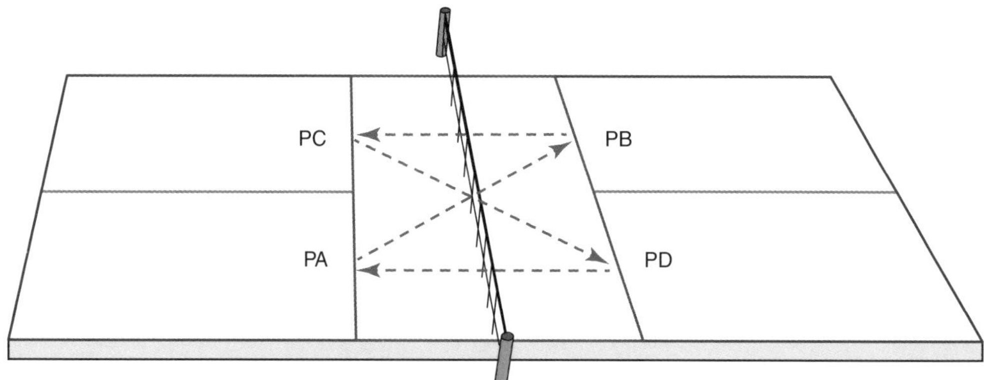

Figure 2.11 Four-player rally at the net drill.

RALLY FROM MIDCOURT

Four players (PA, PB, PC, and PD) take up positions at midcourt; players A and D setting up directly across from one another and players B and C doing the same. Player A bounces the ball and hits it to player B; player B lets the ball bounce once and then hits it to player C; player C lets the ball bounce once and hits it to player D, who lets the ball bounce once and sends it back to player A (figure 2.12). Players keep the rally going as long as possible, each attempting to hit the ball in a controlled manner to the next. The four players rotate counterclockwise, and player A starts the rally again. The rotation process continues until each player has played in each position.

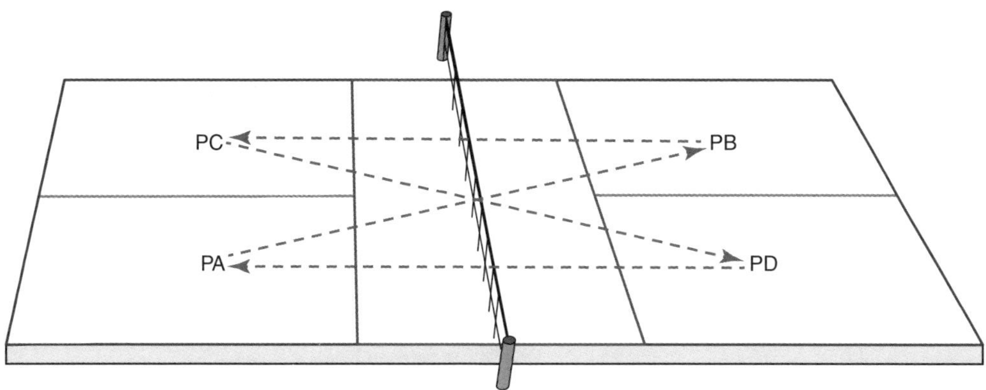

Figure 2.12 Four-player rally from midcourt drill.

SINGLE-PLAYER WALL BALL

Another excellent way to practice seeing the ball contact the paddle is to stand 6 to 12 feet (about 2 to 3 meters) from a wall or backboard and hit the ball against the wall off a bounce, first from your dominant side and then from your nondominant side, as many times as you can (figure 2.13). The surface of the object that you're hitting the ball against will determine how far you can stand from the wall. Because a pickleball is plastic, it won't rebound off the wall as far as a tennis ball or similar type of ball would. Alternatively, you could stand closer than 6 feet from the wall and hit the ball in the air as many times as possible without losing control of the hit.

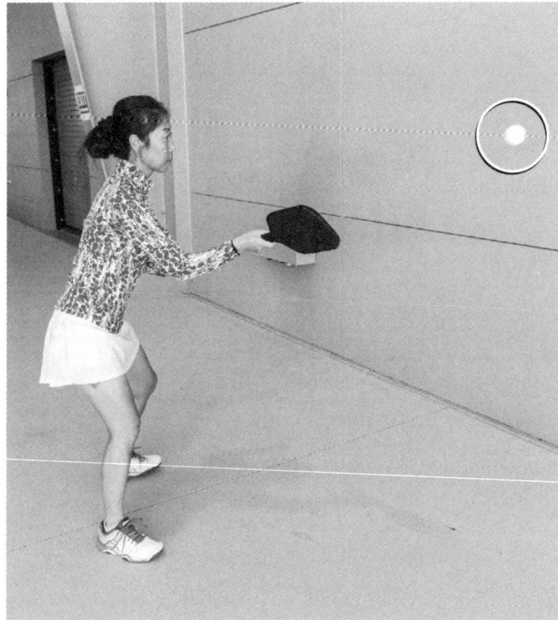

Figure 2.13 Single-player wall ball drill.

ORGANIZING AND RUNNING DRILLS FOR A GROUP

Experienced pickleball players may find themselves in the position of bringing other players along in their development, whether through official coaching duties or simply getting a group together to prepare for an upcoming tournament. As you prepare to organize and run pickleball drills, it's helpful if you have the answers to the following questions:

- How many courts do you have available for drill practice?
- How many participants do you have, and what are their skill levels?
- Do you have the use of a ball hopper or other container to hold balls on each court?
- Do you have the assistance of at least one person per court to help run the drills?
- Any of these drills can be modified for group use. Be creative and keep it fun.

The person helping to run the drills should be someone who has some experience playing pickleball and the ability to throw the ball with some consistency. Here are other considerations:

- Start with something simple and gradually move to more difficult drills. Nothing motivates a new player more than being successful and being told, "Good job!"
- Keep as many players as possible busy. If you have eight players in the group and only four will be practicing the required skills, use the other four to shag balls (that is, chase down the hit balls and return them to the ball hopper). Then after some time, have the two groups switch.
- Always look for something positive to say, even if the player trying the drill is poorly coordinated. Here are examples: "It's okay! You'll do it the next time." "That was the right idea—you're getting it!"
- It doesn't matter what the age or personality of the participant is—no one appreciates being ridiculed or embarrassed. Always try to put every player who is learning the game in a situation that allows for success. If a player is poorly coordinated but still enthusiastic about learning how to play pickleball, place them in a drill situation that they can handle with dignity, even if it's as simple a task as saying "go" or numbering the players to organize into groups.

- You can efficiently split up a large group into smaller workable groups. Say that you have two courts to use and 24 participants, and the participants are all at about the same skill level. Have them stand in a line and number off by 4s. Send the 1s and 2s to court 1 and the 3s and 4s to court 2. The 1s will actually be doing the drill while the 2s become shaggers (they chase down the balls that are hit and replace them in the hopper). On court 2, the 3s become the participants and the 4s are the shaggers. After every participant in that group has had several tries at executing the skill, switch the groups. If the total group is made up of two different skill groups, put one skill group on each court.
- Without singling out or putting pressure on a player who might be struggling, try to not rotate to the next player in line until the player attempting the drill executes a good shot. Always finish on a positive note.
- The leader or teacher of the drill should be directing (explaining and sometimes demonstrating) but should not be in the spotlight! Always be positive with encouraging words for every participant.

Match Point

The importance of controlling and varying the speed and direction of the ball as it is contacted and then leaves the paddle can't be emphasized enough. If you really focus on accomplishing the goal of the drills—hitting the ball in a controlled manner—it will contribute to your ability to execute all the skills and make you a better player.

CHAPTER

3

The Basics: Forehand and Backhand

Forehands and backhands are the two basic strokes used to hit the ball. When a player returns a ball that has bounced from a position midcourt to deep in the court, including the return of a serve, the backhand or forehand is often called a "groundstroke." If the ball is hit before it bounces, it is termed a "volley." Volleys have extra importance in pickleball, due to the presence of the non-volley zone (NVZ), often called the "kitchen," so chapter 5 is devoted to them. Both forehands and backhands can be groundstrokes or volleys depending on whether the ball has already bounced or not.

A forehand is struck from the same side of your body as your dominant hand (the hand with which you hold the paddle), and a backhand is hit from the opposite side, with the paddle reaching across the body. When the ball is coming to you from across the net, you should be in a good ready position, as explained in chapter 2. Hold the paddle in front of your body in a relaxed position in preparation for executing either a forehand or backhand shot. You should feel light on your feet, shift your weight somewhat toward your toes, and be ready to move quickly in any direction.

The success of your forehand or backhand is directly related to your ability to move in all directions on the court—right, left, forward, and backward—quickly and smoothly. Your distance from the bouncing ball determines the type, length, and number of steps required for moving into the best position from which to return it. If the ball is coming close to you, take small steps to adjust your position; if the ball bounces farther from you, you will have to stride more quickly or run to it. It's highly important to have a correct finishing position in relation to the ball and a balanced and controlled stance.

You Can Do It

FOREHAND GROUNDSTROKE

From the moment the ball leaves the opponent's paddle, you should be tracking its flight with your eyes to judge its speed and direction. As quickly as you can, move to where the ball is traveling, to be ready for your shot before the ball arrives. At that point, you should assume a position that is partially facing the net and partially facing the nearest sideline, with your weight balanced over your feet (figure 3.1). The bouncing ball should be between you and the net and on your paddle-arm side.

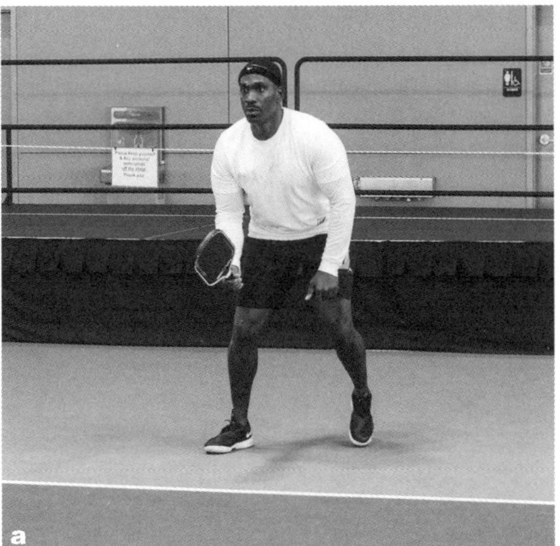

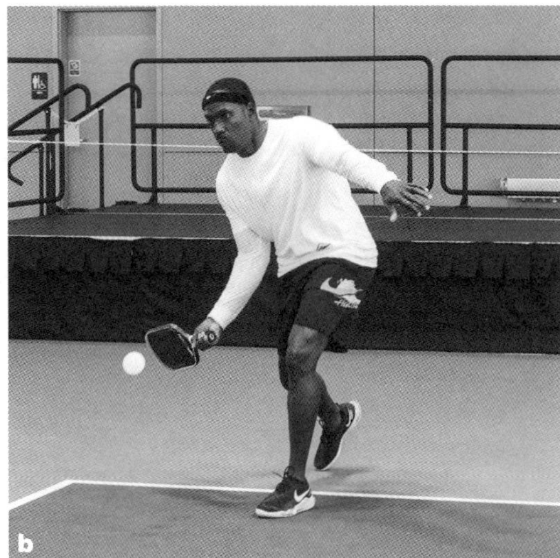

Figure 3.1 Moving into position for a forehand groundstroke.

As you're moving into position, draw your paddle arm back in preparation for the forward arm swing. With your weight on your rear foot (the right foot if you're right-handed), swing your paddle arm backward while keeping it parallel to the ground (figure 3.2*a*). Shift your weight from your rear foot to your front foot and tighten your grip on the paddle somewhat as you contact the ball at a point just off your front knee (3.2*b*). A firm but not too tight grip allows for better control of the paddle and puts more force on the hit. Follow through by allowing your swinging arm to continue through toward the target (3.2*c*).

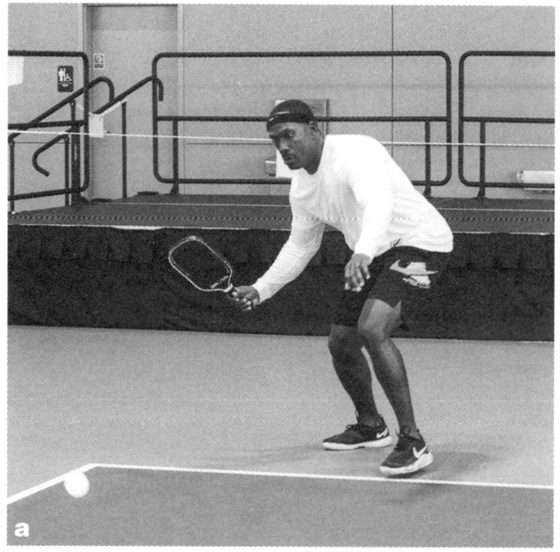

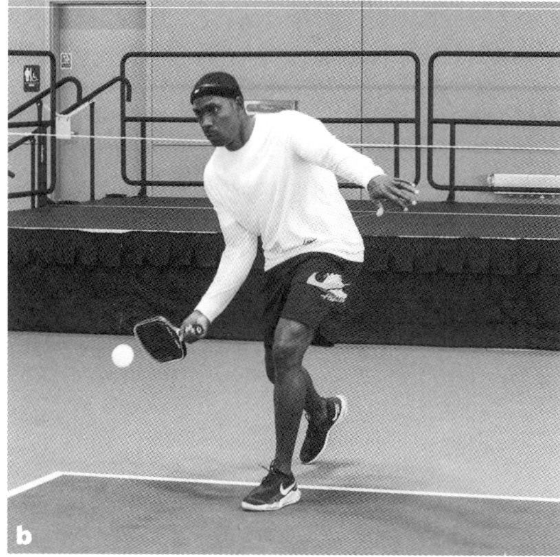

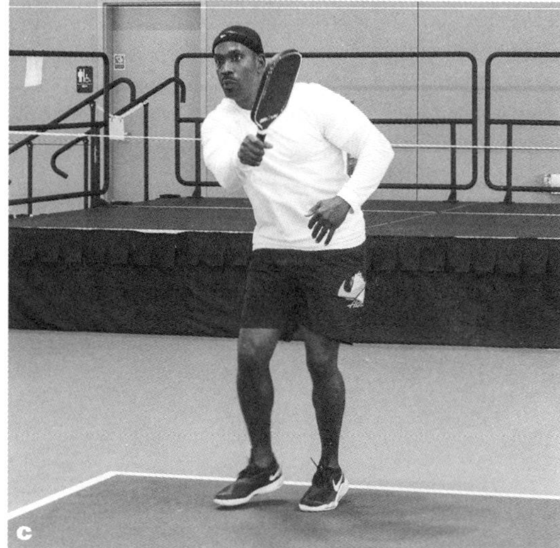

Figure 3.2 Forehand groundstroke: (*a*) preparing for the forward swing, (*b*) contact, and (*c*) follow-through.

BACKHAND GROUNDSTROKE

The same principles apply when you're hitting a backhand groundstroke except that you move to the side opposite your paddle hand. While some players change the grip on the paddle by rotating the paddle slightly to the right or clockwise (for a right-handed player), others do not. It's a matter of personal preference. Pivot toward your left side and take short, controlled steps toward the oncoming ball. Move to a position that is behind and to the side of the anticipated bounce of the ball. Take the paddle back by moving it back across your body (figure 3.3*a*). With your weight on your rear foot, swing your paddle arm forward, keeping

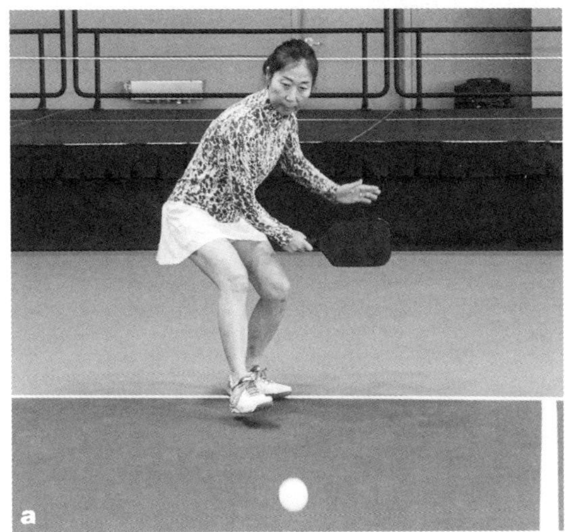

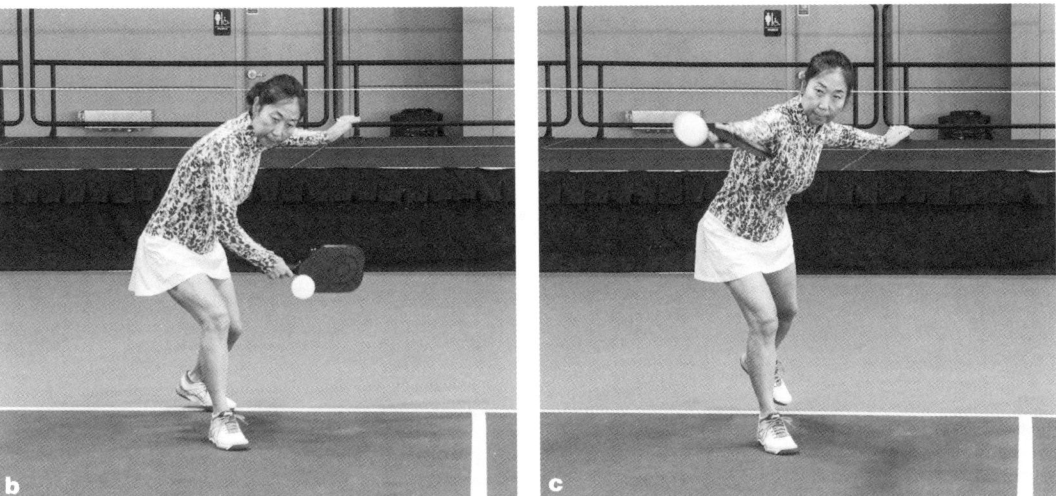

Figure 3.3 Backhand groundstroke: (*a*) beginning of the backward swing, (*b*) contact, and (*c*) follow-through.

the face of the paddle perpendicular to the ground. Contact the ball between your body and the net and off your front knee (the right one, for a right-hander) (3.3*b*). After contact, follow through toward the target (3.3*c*). Figure 3.4 shows the two-handed backhand groundstroke.

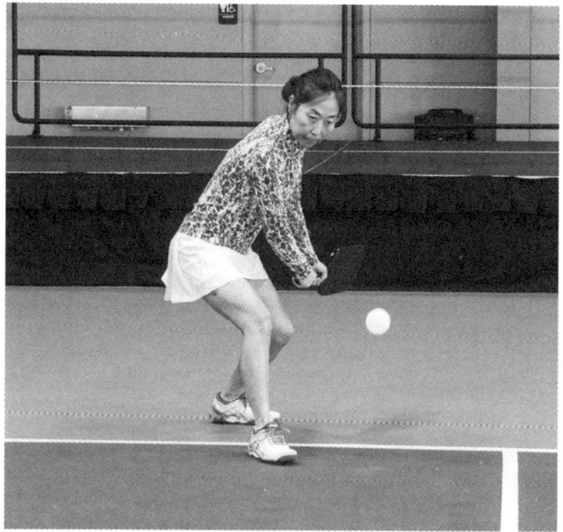

Figure 3.4 Two-handed backhand groundstroke.

More to Choose and Use

PUTTING SPIN ON THE BALL

After you feel confident hitting both your forehand and backhand strokes normally (figure 3.5*a*), you might want to experiment with putting some spin on the ball. If you are just learning pickleball, it's best to focus on hitting shots consistently with control before concentrating on spin. However, some players find it more natural to hit certain shots with spin. If it's easier for you to hit a backhand with some slice (sidespin) or a forehand with topspin, great. Just don't sacrifice the goal of hitting each shot accurately and consistently for the sake of adding spin.

The three types of spin that can be applied to the ball are topspin, backspin, and sidespin (or slice).

To put topspin on the ball, at the point of contact you should sweep the paddle head upward on the ball, scuffing the paddle face across the back surface of the ball rather than striking it squarely (3.5*b*). The ball will dip downward sooner than a flat-struck ball. Upon contact with the ground, it will bounce higher and scoot away from the net. Many players place topspin on the ball when using a forehand groundstroke as the ball can be driven harder while staying in bounds, dipping down to make the opponent's return more difficult and keeping the bounce inside the baseline and sidelines.

Backspin on the ball involves swiping the ball downward, with a slightly open paddle face as you are contacting it (3.5*c*). A ball with backspin will sail farther than one with topspin, bounce lower and shorter, and can

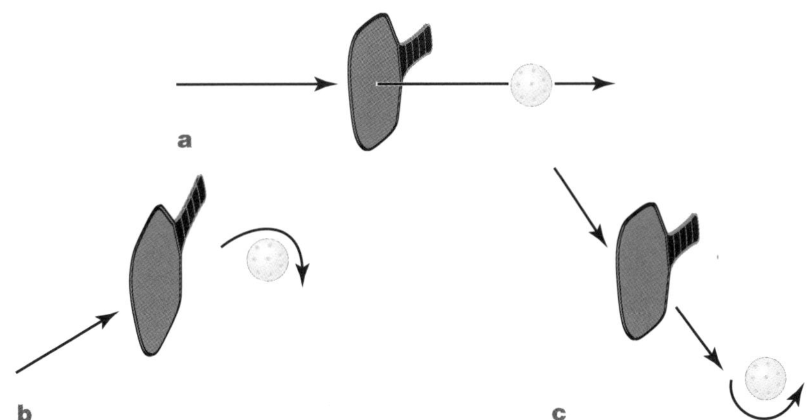

Figure 3.5 Action of the paddle on the ball for (*a*) a stroke without spin, (*b*) a stroke with topspin, and (*c*) a stroke with backspin.

even travel back toward the net upon contact with the ground. Backspin can be especially effective with a forehand or backhand stroke that is just hard enough to drop the spinning ball over the net.

Applying sidespin, or slice, requires moving the paddle either from left to right or from right to left as you contact the ball. A shot with sidespin can visibly curve in flight; then, upon contact with the ground, the ball will hop even further in that direction, either to the right or to the left, depending on how you hit it. When a right-handed player hits a backhand serve or groundstroke, it is common to put a natural left-to-right sidespin on the ball, which causes the ball to bounce away from the forehand of a right-handed receiving player.

Although placing spin on the ball makes it more difficult for your opponent to return the ball, it can be difficult to control. To be a good pickleball player, most new players should be comfortable hitting the basic shots using a flat contact of the ball before striving to add extra spin to their game.

While practicing the forehand and backhand groundstrokes, keep in mind that because a pickleball is plastic and has holes in it, the ball won't bounce as high or travel as far as a solid ball, such as a tennis ball, would. This means that you have to move to the ball; the ball won't come to you! It may take some time for you to get a feel for how close to the ball you need to be to execute a solid forehand or backhand groundstroke, but don't get discouraged. The more times you practice it, the easier it becomes. Most important is that as you contact the ball, you should be far enough from it to allow your paddle arm to move freely so that your arm is not cramped, and the ball contacts the paddle at the center of the face (known as the sweet spot).

Ignoring any spin, the trajectory of the oncoming ball before the actual bounce will determine the height of the bounce. A lofted ball will bounce higher than a low, hard-driven ball. Being able to anticipate the height of the bounce will assist you in planning your next move. Ideally, when executing a groundstroke, you should contact the ball between the moment of impact with the court and the peak of the bounce (figure 3.6). Contacting the ball before it peaks allows you to return the ball more quickly than if you wait to contact it after it peaks and is on the way back down. In general, a shot returned more quickly—whether it is a dink or drive, volley or groundstroke—is more likely to reach an opponent before they are ready.

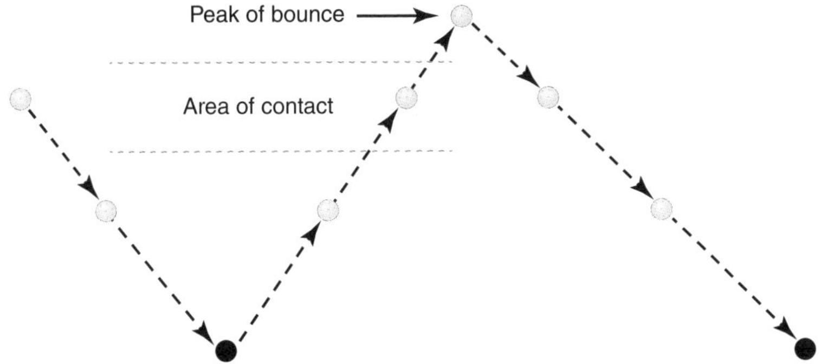

Figure 3.6 Anticipate and strike ahead of the peak of the bounce.

Take It to the Court

Identify any error that might cause your forehand or backhand stroke to be erratic. Recognize the error and be able to correct it so that you can become a better player. Here are some examples of common errors and tips for correcting them.

Not making solid contact with the ball

- *Keep your eye on the ball.* See the ball not only hit the paddle but also leave the face of the paddle. An aid for practicing this is to mark a colored ring on the ball or a colored ring around the center of the ball. The player hitting the ball calls out the color of the ring.
- *Focus on using a controlled backswing and a follow-through.* As you see the ball coming toward you, take the paddle back (but not up over your shoulders) in preparation for the forward swing. After contacting the ball, follow through with your paddle arm in the direction of the intended flight of the ball. Concentrate on using a controlled backswing and follow-through every time you hit the ball using a forehand or backhand groundstroke. Because of the small size of a pickleball court and the lightweight ball, the backswing and follow-through should be less exaggerated than a tennis swing, with the paddle in front of your body in the "ready" position as much as possible to allow for quick reactions.
- *Contact the ball on the sweet spot of the paddle face.* To do this, you must exaggerate seeing the ball actually contact the face of the paddle. You might even draw a circle in chalk on the face of your paddle to define the sweet spot.
- *Consciously firm up your grip on the paddle at the time of contact with the ball.* A loose grip will deaden the force applied to the ball, a skill we will discuss later. On the other hand, don't use a "death grip" squeeze either. A firm grip is roughly a 7 out of 10.

Hitting the ball too long so it goes out of bounds over the baseline

- *Concentrate on keeping the face of the paddle in a square position or perpendicular to the ground when contacting the ball.* If the face of the paddle is open, the ball coming off the paddle face will travel upward. Combined with a forceful swing, it will cause the ball to go too high and too long.
- *Focus on using a controlled swing that is parallel to the ground rather than hitting the ball as hard as you can.* If you are too forceful and aggressive as you hit the ball and the forward

swing of your paddle arm is upward, the ball will travel high and deep—probably too deep!

Hitting the ball into the net

- *Ideally, try to move into a position where you can contact the ball at the same point in the bounce using a swing that is parallel to the ground, at approximately the same height as your flexed knees.* Controlling the speed of the swing and being consistent in timing your swing to the bouncing ball are important for successful hits.
- *Be sure that the face of the paddle is square or slightly open at the point of ball contact.*
- *Focus on bending your knees and going down to the ball if the bounce is low and the ball is close to the ground.* If this is the case, the forward swing of your paddle arm needs to be upward, so the ball can travel high enough to clear the net.
- *Control your arm swing and think of directing the ball to a strategic spot in the opposing court rather than hitting the ball as hard as you can.*

Consistently hitting the ball too far to the nondominant side of your body, causing it to go out of bounds over that sideline

- *Focus on moving to a spot behind and to the side of the bouncing ball.* Proper body position allows the paddle face to be square to the net when you make contact with the ball (figure 3.7). If the ball is too far in front of your body when you make ball contact, the paddle will face the sideline of your nondominant side, causing the ball to go out of bounds in that direction.
- *A firm grip on the paddle contributes to a controlled hit.*

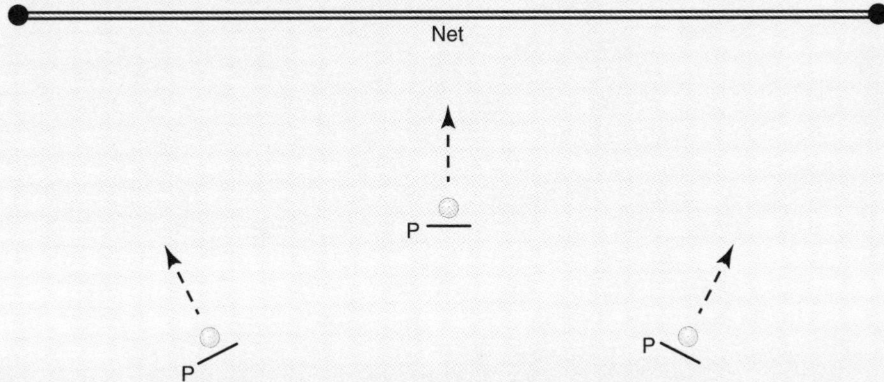

Figure 3.7 For maximum control, get into position slightly behind and beside the ball and square the paddle face to the net.

Consistently hitting the ball too far to the dominant side of your body, causing it to go out of bounds over the sideline

- *Be sure that your body position just before contacting the ball is behind and to the side of the ball.* Proper positioning allows the face of the paddle at the moment of ball contact to be square to the net. If the ball is closer to your rear foot than your forward foot when you make contact, the paddle will face that sideline, causing the ball to go out of bounds.
- *Grip the paddle firmly (without squeezing) as you contact the ball.* A too-loose grip will cause the flight of the ball to be erratic.

Make in-game adjustments rather than allow yourself to commit the same error repeatedly. If you hit two consecutive shots into the net, tell yourself that something has to change. On the next play, exaggerate the correction of the error. Chances are that the ball will go over the net and land inbounds. If you consistently miss your groundstrokes to the left, aim to the extreme right. If you then miss to the right, adjust your point of aim closer to the center line. Follow this procedure until you are able to zero in and put the ball where you want it.

Give It a Go

Trying to correct errors in the execution of a skill is nearly impossible during a game. It requires repetitive practice of the skill in a controlled situation. As you complete each of the following drills, focus on executing the skill correctly every time.

SOFT TOSS

The feeder (F) uses a soft underhand movement to toss the ball to the hitter (P) (figure 3.8). F tosses the ball to the forehand side of P, who hits the tossed ball after the bounce using a forehand groundstroke. The feeder tosses the next ball to the backhand side of P, and P hits the tossed ball after the bounce using a backhand groundstroke. After some time, players switch roles so that F becomes the new P and the former P is now alternating ball tosses to the new P's forehand and backhand.

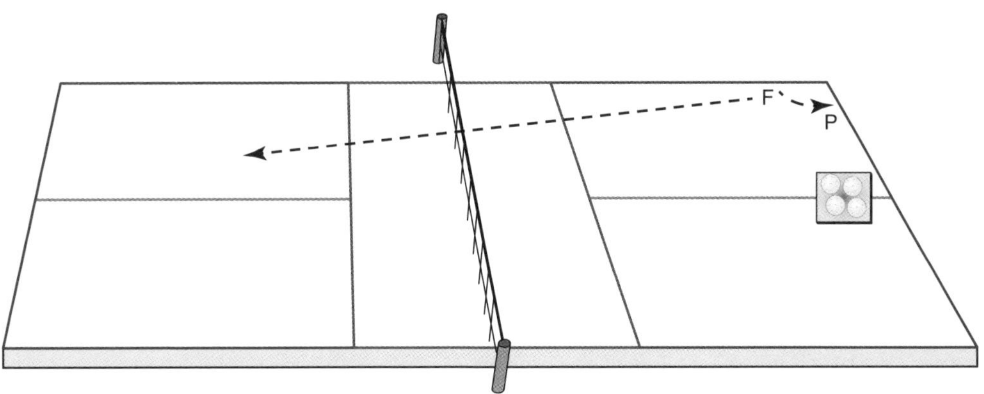

Figure 3.8 Soft toss drill.

HIT OFF A THROW

This drill is an extension of the Soft Toss Drill. This time the feeder F will be on the opposite side of the net from the player P. The feeder F throws a slightly lofted ball across the net, aiming to have the ball bounce in front of P and to their forehand side. The player returns the ball over the net using a forehand groundstroke (figure 3.9). After three or four hits, the feeder throws the next few to the backhand side. The player will aim to return the backhands over the net. After the player has had a chance to hit ten or so groundstrokes, both forehand and backhand, the player becomes the feeder and the previous feeder has their chance to practice their groundstrokes from both sides of the body. This drill can also be used by alternating forehands and backhands on each throw. As always, players should practice returning to their ready position after each shot.

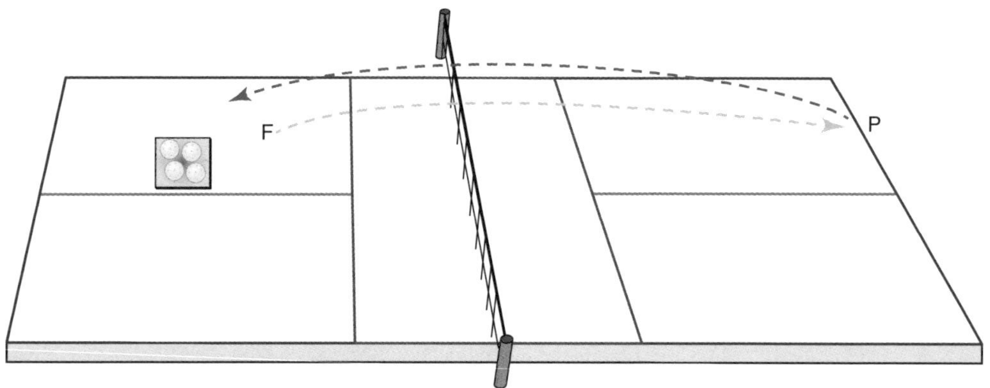

Figure 3.9 Hit off a throw drill.

RALLY FROM THE BASELINE

Players set up near the baseline, one on each end of the court, and rally across the net using one ball, much as they would in a match. The players attempt to keep the rally going as long as possible. Strive to hit the shots so that they bounce on the court, allowing your drill partner to return it with a groundstroke. Make sure to practice hitting shots with both forehands and backhands, since beginning players often favor one side or the other and a well-rounded player needs confidence in both. This drill can also be done with two players on each side of the net (four players total), much like a game of doubles pickleball (figure 3.10).

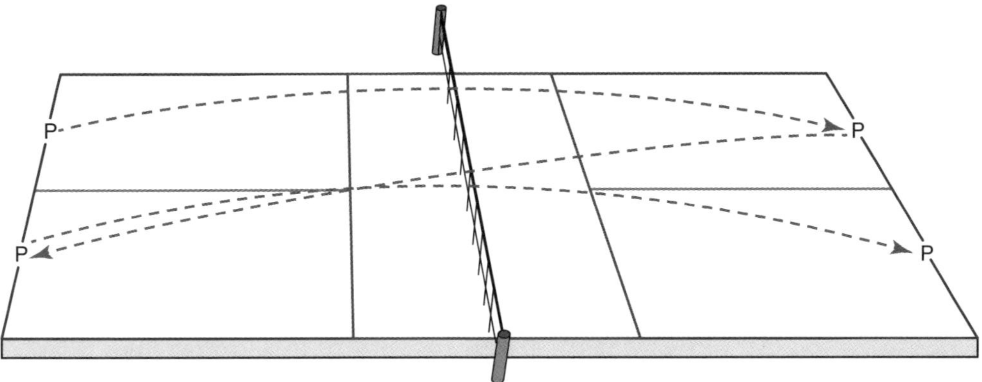

Figure 3.10 Four-player rally from the baseline drill.

Match Point

The phrase "more games are lost than are won" is absolutely true! So often in competition, it is the team that commits fewer unforced errors that ends up winning the game. Many players and doubles teams allow themselves to commit error after error with no noticeable attempt to change how or what they're doing, except to try more and more difficult "winner" shots. The net and "out" lines, not the opponents, have become their worst enemy! Don't let this happen to you. From the first time you hold a paddle and throughout your pickleball playing days, make it a primary goal to keep the ball in play, giving your opponent another chance to make their own unforced error.

CHAPTER

4

Serve and Return

The serve puts the ball in play. If the server doesn't get the serve in legally, the rally is over without the opponent needing to do anything. Because of that, the serve could be considered the most important pickleball skill to master. You don't have to serve hard, but you do need to be able to hit the ball legally from a position behind your baseline over the net into the opponent's service court, which is diagonally opposite you.

Perhaps the second most important skill of a game is the return of serve. Like the serve itself, it is an uncontested shot—neither can be returned with an aggressive shot hit in the air (a volley) because the ball must bounce before it is hit. Therefore, both the serve and return of serve should be two of your most consistent, practiced shots.

The rules for a legal serve continue to evolve. The "drop serve" option is a newer rule that simplifies learning the serve for many new players. Always practice and play following the most recent iterations of the rules.

If the serve is hit before the ball bounces (the original serve), other rules apply: contact must be made below the waist, the arm must be moving in an upward arc, and the paddle head, defined as the part of the paddle excluding the handle, cannot be above any part of the line formed where the wrist joint bends. If the ball is released by the hand and allowed to bounce before being struck (the "drop serve"), the rules about the waist, upward motion, and position of the paddle head do not apply. This release ("drop") of the ball must be done without adding any spin or tossing it in any way.

You Can Do It

FOREHAND SERVE
FOR A RIGHT-HANDED PLAYER

Most commonly used is a forehand drive serve. Stand in a forward stride position behind the baseline with your left shoulder pointing toward the target and your weight on your back foot. The ball is in your left hand, and your left arm is extended toward the net. Bend at the waist slightly, take your paddle arm back, drop or toss the ball between you and the target without adding spin to the ball (figure 4.1*a*), swing your paddle arm forward in an underhand motion, and contact the ball below your waist (4.1*b*). After ball contact, follow through by bringing your arm up and toward the target (4.1*c*), driving the ball deep toward the baseline diagonally across the net from you. Many people describe this underhand swing motion as similar to bowling or tossing a bean bag in cornhole.

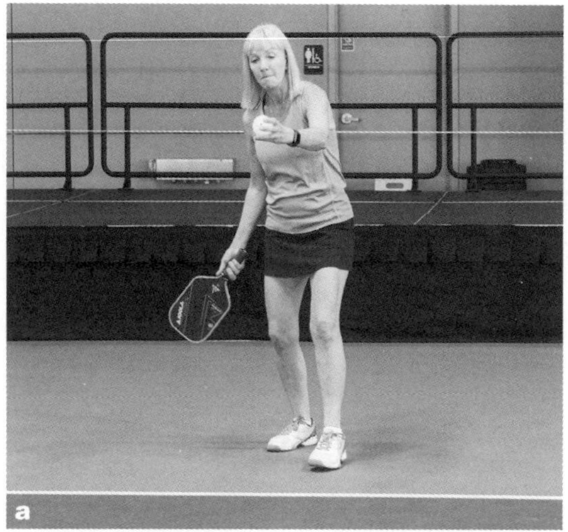

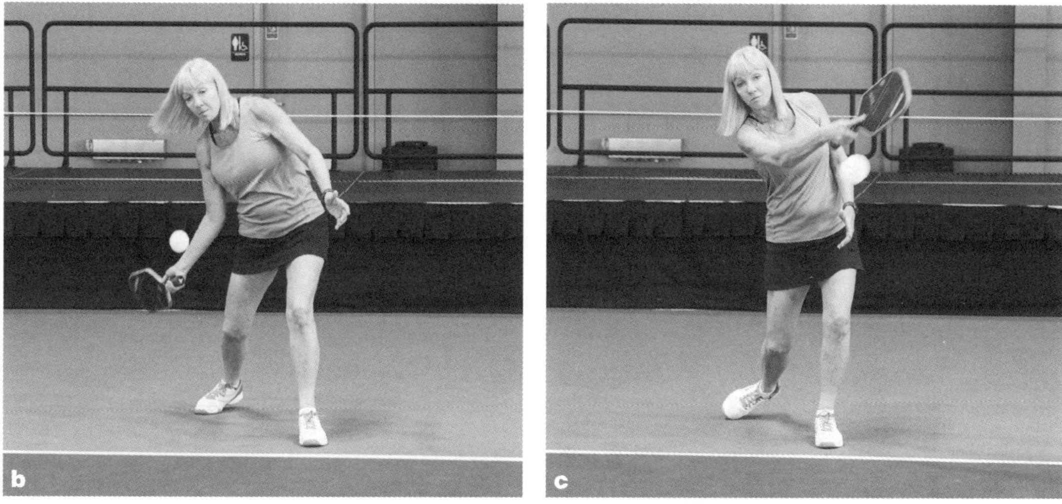

Figure 4.1 The forehand drive serve: (*a*) preparation, (*b*) contact, and (*c*) follow-through.

If you are using the "drop serve" option, be careful to *drop* the ball only; do not add any spin or velocity to it. After the dropped ball bounces, the goal should be to hit the serve near the top of the bounce (figure 4.2). The higher you reach above your head to drop the ball, the higher it bounces. The one time a high drop may hurt is if it is windy enough to blow the dropped ball toward or away from you before you can serve it.

One serve targeting option is a short crosscourt serve that lands just beyond the non-volley line. After a series of deep serves, the opponent will likely not expect a short soft serve, which may lead to an easy point.

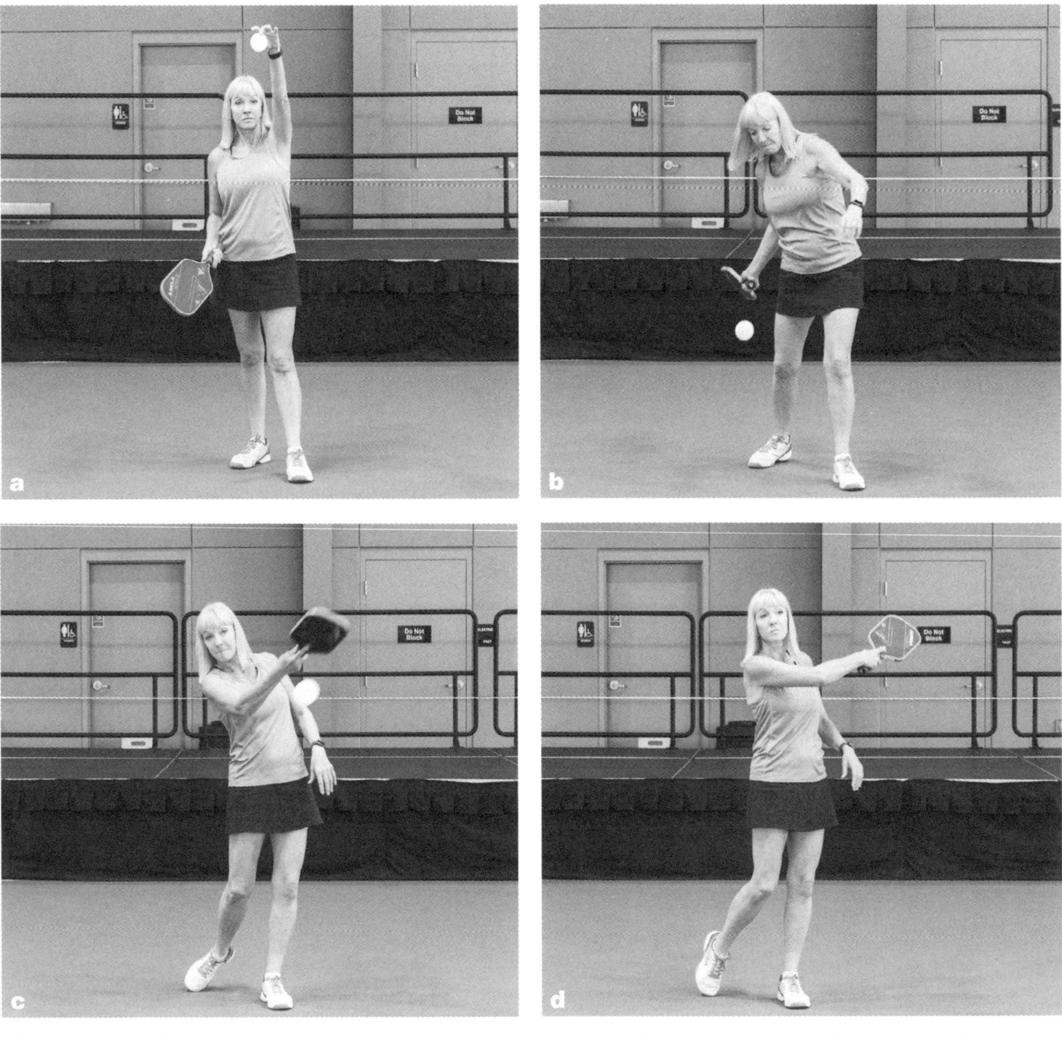

Figure 4.2 The drop serve: *(a)* prepare to release the ball, *(b)* allow the ball to bounce, *(c-d)* contact, and follow through.

A third option for serving and perhaps the easiest to execute is the lob serve. When executing a lob serve, stand in a balanced upright position with your body facing the net and your left foot slightly ahead of the right foot (for the right-handed server). The preparation (figure 4.3*a*) and execution are similar to the drive serve and can be used with or without the drop serve, but the goal is to hit the serve in a high arc that lands deep in the opponent's court. Swing the paddle arm forward and make contact with the face of the paddle behind and below the ball (4.3*b*). Follow through up and toward the target (4.3*c*). Picture the ball being lofted and landing deep in the intended service court. A lob

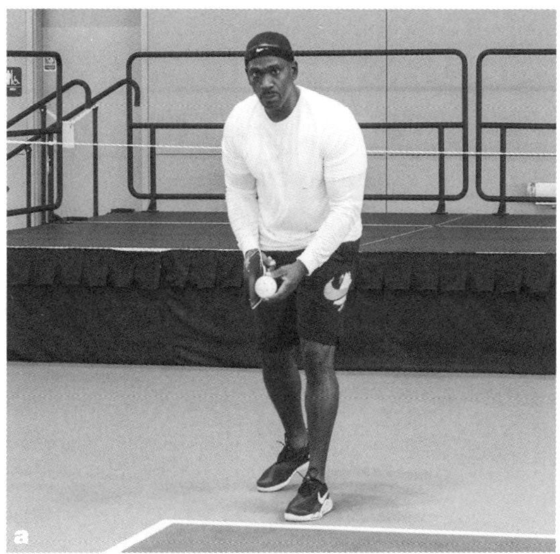

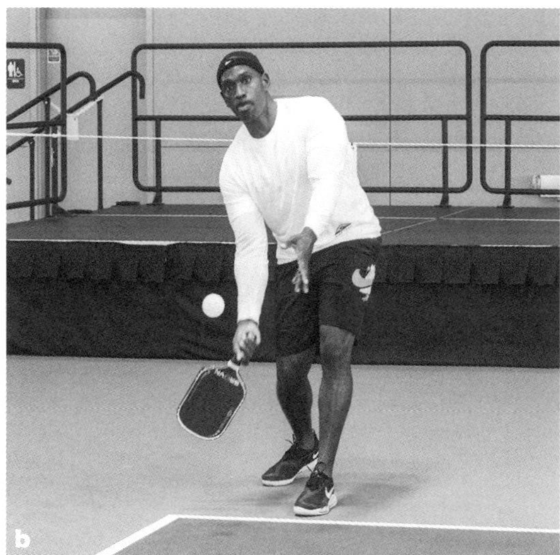

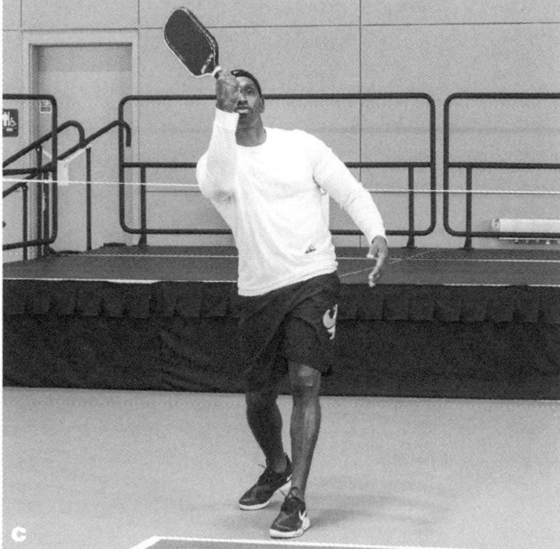

Figure 4.3 The lob serve: (*a*) preparation, (*b*) contact, and (*c*) follow-through.

serve is an excellent serve to mix in with a forehand drive serve. The slow speed of the ball as well as the high bounce often throw off the receiving player's timing.

In summary, the forehand offers several possible choices of serve: a hard-driven serve, a shallow crosscourt serve, and a lofted lob serve, each of which can be done either with or without spin or a dropped bounce before striking the ball. Your decision about which serve to use depends on what motion is most comfortable for you, the position of the player receiving the serve, and (if known) how that player tends to react to each kind of serve.

BACKHAND SERVE FOR A RIGHT-HANDED PLAYER

Players who cannot control the flight of the ball when using a forehand serve may find that a backhand serve works better. Some players who excel in using a forehand serve also find it useful to have the backhand serve in their arsenal. Just as there are variations of the forehand serve, there are variations of the backhand serve. Most common is for a right-handed player to assume a "side-stride" position behind the baseline, with the right side toward the net. The right foot points to a spot between the net and the left sideline (figure 4.4*a*). The ball is in the left hand, and the arms are crossed in front of the body. The ball is dropped in line with the intended target, and the paddle arm swings forward and contacts the ball as it travels downward (4.4*b*). The swinging arm continues in a follow-through motion toward the target (4.4*c*). This serve is easy to execute because only the upper body of the server moves. It is also deceiving to the receiver and difficult to return because of a natural sidespin on the ball. Backhand serves can be hit in any way that forehands can: with spin, lobbed, driven deep, or to the short corner. Many players find that using the drop serve to let the ball bounce before contact makes the backhand serve motion much easier to control and repeat consistently.

How you serve the ball and how you look while serving are incidental as long as you serve legally and successfully. Try several methods of serving until you find one or more that work for you.

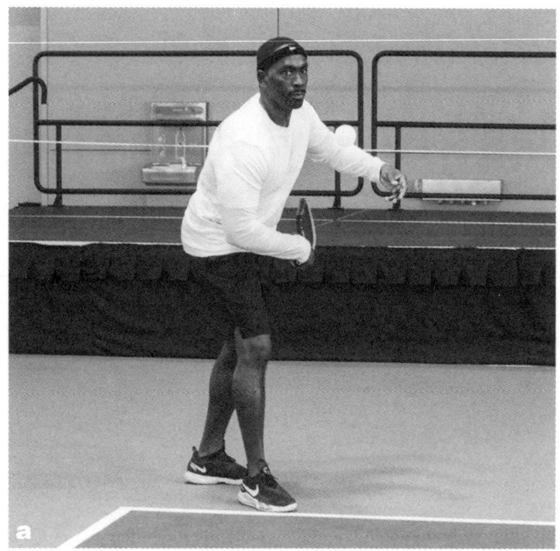

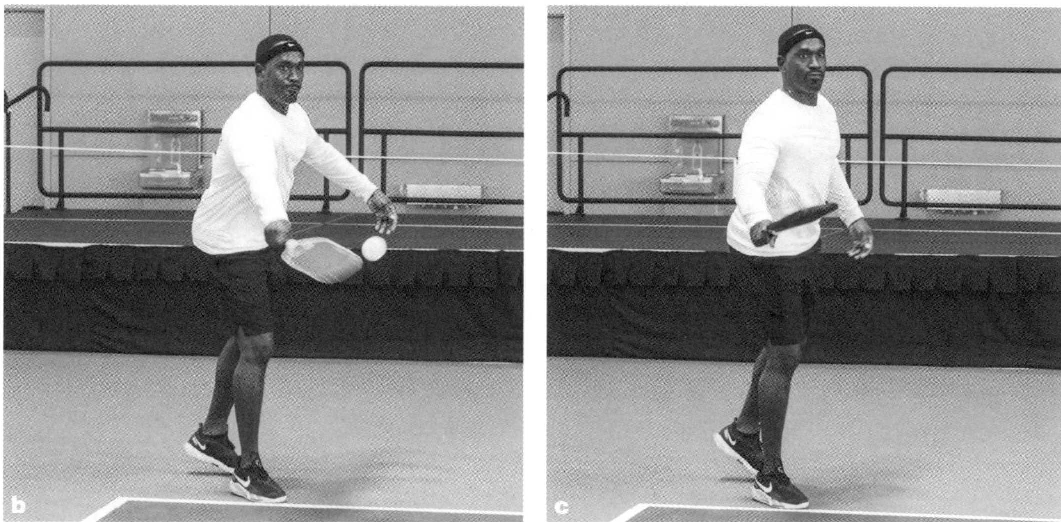

Figure 4.4 The backhand serve: (*a*) preparation, (*b*) contact, and (*c*) follow-through.

More to Choose and Use

OBJECTIVES AND STRATEGIES FOR SERVE AND RETURN

While the serve may be the most important shot in pickleball to master, it is also one of the easiest. It can be hit with a forehand or backhand and the ball can be dropped from the hand and either hit in the air or allowed to bounce before it is struck. The rules pertaining to the serve are changed or clarified periodically in an attempt to standardize the serving motion and to eliminate the possibility of a player gaining an unfair advantage while serving.

If the serve is hit before the ball bounces (the original serve), other rules apply: contact must be made below the waist, the arm "must be moving in an upward arc," and the paddle head, defined as the part of the paddle excluding the handle, "cannot be above any part of the line formed where the wrist joint bends." If the ball is released by the hand and allowed to bounce before being struck (the drop serve), the rules about the waist, upward motion, and position of the paddle head do not apply.

Most important among the rules concerning the serve are that the ball must be served from behind the baseline, clear the net, and land in the opponent's service box (diagonally opposite the server). If any part of the ball contacts the non-volley zone (NVZ) line or any other part of the NVZ, it is a fault. All other lines of the service box are considered to be inbounds. If the served ball clips the net but lands in the proper court afterward, the ball is in play and must be returned after the first bounce.

You need to understand the "double-bounce rule" in order to understand the strategies involved in serving and returning the serve. Essentially, the rule is that each side must make one groundstroke (one bounce on the serve and one bounce on the return, totaling the "double" bounce) before the ball can be volleyed. Because of this rule, neither the serve nor the return of serve can be countered with an offensive volley shot wherein the ball is contacted with force in the air and angled sharply down. Without the worry that your serve or return of serve might be smashed back for a winner, you should execute both of these shots with consistency and success.

The trajectory of the served ball can be hard driven and low over the net or it can be a slow-moving lofted shot (figure 4.5). The goal of the server should be to consistently serve balls that land in the back 3 to 4 feet (a meter or a bit more) of the opponent's service court (figure 4.6). Because of the double-bounce rule, the ball must bounce once before the opponent can return it. Therefore, a served ball that lands deep in the court keeps the receiver deep in their court and far from the net, which is a defensive position. The farther from the net that the player contacts the ball, the more time it takes the player to make the next strategic move, which is to the NVZ line.

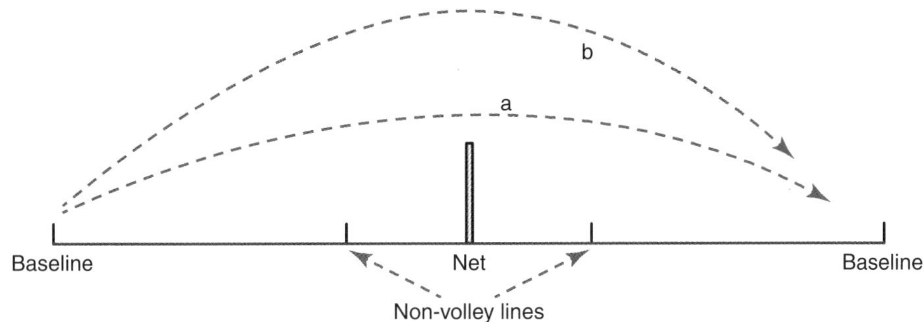

Figure 4.5 Flight paths of (*a*) a hard-driven serve and (*b*) a lob serve.

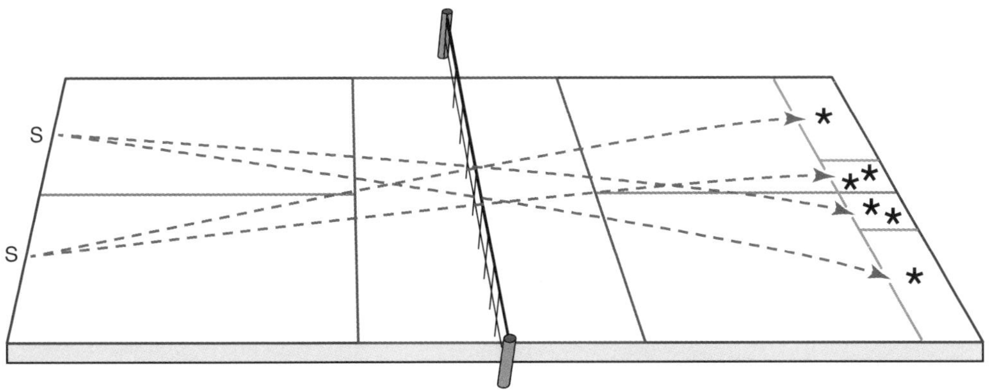

Figure 4.6 Servers attempting to hit target areas for good (*) and excellent (**) serves.

SERVE POSITION

When you play doubles, your position behind the baseline when serving depends somewhat on the type of serve that you plan to use. However, it's not wise to vary your position too much because it will telegraph to your opponents the type of serve that you plan to use. For example, if your intent is to hit a short crosscourt serve, you can get more of an angle on the hit ball if you stand close to the sideline rather than in the center of the court. Other than that, you should maintain a position behind your baseline in a position that enables you to cover your half of the court on the return of the serve.

When you play singles, the strongest position for serving is close to the center line. This puts you in a strong position from which to move to the right or the left to get to the return shot.

RETURN

The partner of the player returning the serve (R2) stands behind the non-volley line, and the player preparing to return the serve (R1) stands deep in or behind the service court, ready to return the ball (figure 4.7).

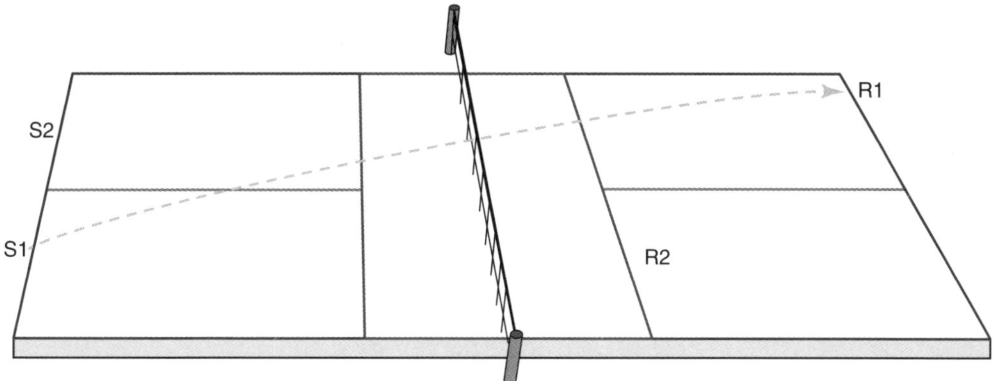

Figure 4.7 Players in position for receiving the serve.

Both R1 and R2 should appear alert and ready for the next play. As the serve travels over the net, R1 moves to a position in relation to the anticipated bounce of the ball that allows them to return it with a soft forehand groundstroke. R1's goal is to return the ball slow and deep into the backhand corner of the opponent's court (figure 4.8). It should be slow and deep to give the player returning the serve (R1) time to get to the non-volley line and get set for the next play and to keep the serving team deep in their court. They must let the ball bounce once before they can hit the ball in the air, a shot usually executed from the non-volley line that can be offensive in nature.

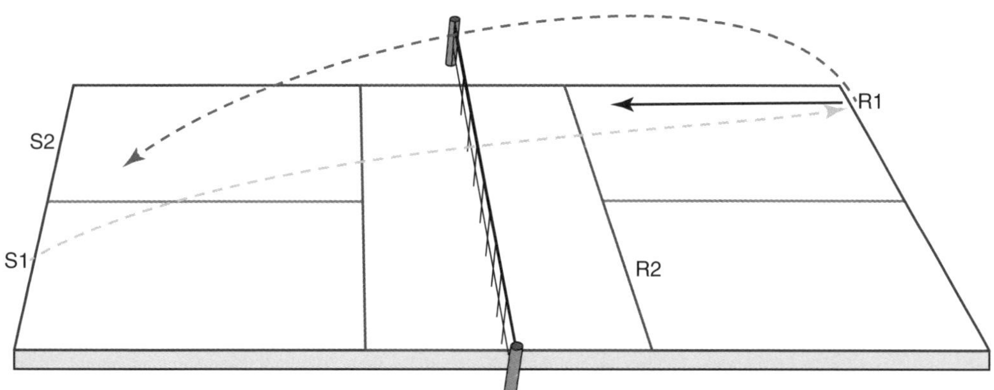

Figure 4.8 Returning the serve to the backhand corner and moving up to the line.

The second choice of a target on the return of serve is for the ball to be returned slow and deep down the middle of the opponent's court (figure 4.9). This is especially effective when returning the serve from behind the left service court. Immediately after executing the return of serve, the player should move forward to a position at the non-volley line alongside their partner. The ideal position for a doubles team is side by side at the net because it is an offensive position. From this location they can cut off balls quickly.

The receiving team (R1 and R2) is now at the net (behind the non-volley line) while the serving team (S1 and S2) is still deep in their court. Players on the serving team must stay back because the returned ball must bounce once before they can return it. If either player were to go forward to the non-volley line and then return the ball while it was still in the air, that player would be in violation of the double-bounce rule, and a fault would be charged. With both players at the net, the receiving team has the advantage. Therefore, at this point, the serving team would try to execute a shot that would enable them to get to the net. (These shots are explained in later chapters.)

In singles play, the strongest return of serve is typically down the line on the backhand side of the server. If, by chance, the server's backhand is stronger than the forehand, hit the ball down the line but to the forehand side.

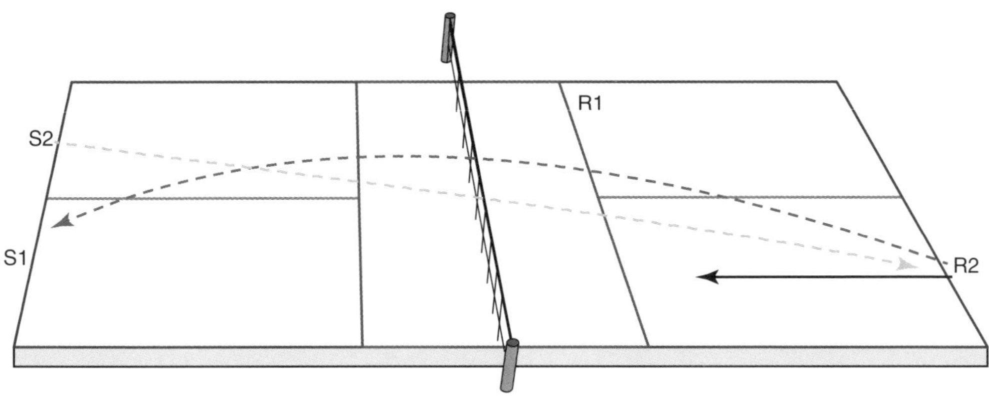

Figure 4.9 Returning the serve down the middle and moving up to the line.

Take It to the Court

The ability to recognize errors in serving and returning the serve and to correct them is a definite advantage. If you do commit an error, think about it and work on it between games. Here are some common errors and tips for correcting them.

Hitting the ball into the net

- *Concentrate on swinging the paddle forward and through the ball sooner.* Follow through slightly up and in the direction of the desired flight of the ball.
- *Focus on dropping or tossing the ball consistently.* Unless you are purposely trying a different serve, such as a short angled one into the corner, the toss or drop of the ball and the subsequent contact of the ball need to be the same every time.
- *On the follow-through, be sure that the face of the paddle is facing up.*
- *Keep your eye on the ball when striking it. Looking up too early will cause it to hit the net or land short.*

Serving too long

- *Focus on bending at the waist and bending the knees as you prepare the forward swing.*
- *Controlling the hit is more important than hitting the ball too hard.*
- *If your normal serve is a hard one and there is some space behind the baseline, assume your starting position a few steps back from the baseline.*
- *Emphasize the forward motion of the swing to drive the ball, versus more upward motion, which can send the ball long.*

Missing the serve to the right or to the left

- *Be sure that your grip is firm so that the paddle doesn't turn in your hand as you contact the ball.*
- *Be sure that the face of the paddle is moving toward the desired target at all times.*
- *Be sure that the drop or toss of the ball is in line with the intended target.*

Returning the serve too shallow, allowing the serving team to get to the net

- *Focus on hitting the served ball more forcefully as well as on a path that easily clears the top of the net.*
- *Exaggerate how deep you hit a lofted shot. If your returns start going too long, you can then dial back the force of your return while keeping the loft.*

The idea is to serve the ball *exactly the same way every time*, unless you are purposely varying it based on your knowledge of the returner. Don't change the way you toss or drop the ball, take the paddle back, or swing your arm forward! You *can* vary where you stand behind the baseline before serving, and you *can* turn your body slightly to one side or the other. But the actual movement of your body parts while serving should be consistent and repeatable on your serves. Once you have adopted at least one method of serving that feels comfortable and results in a serve that travels over the net and lands deep in the appropriate court, strive for accuracy and consistency every time you step onto the pickleball court.

What if your regular serve seems "off" (i.e., for some inexplicable reason you start missing your serves)? You may get frustrated and try even harder, but the balls still will not go over the net and land inbounds. If this happens, it's good to have a secondary (backup) serve that you can use until you get your old serve back. If you usually serve the ball low and hard, try a lob serve. Stand in a fairly upright position, drop the ball in line with the target, and swing underhand as if you are lobbing the ball. Another backup serve might be a backhand drop serve (described earlier in this chapter). The method that you use is incidental as long as it is legal, goes over the net, and lands in the proper court. The ability to serve using more than one method can help you relax and enjoy the game.

Give It a Go

The following drills allow you to practice both the serve and the return of serve in a controlled situation. Focus on executing both with 100 percent accuracy. The serving drills are presented first.

SERVE AND CATCH

Four players are on the court in a serving position (S1, S2, S3, and S4). Players S1 and S2 begin with a ball. Players S1 and S3 serve back and forth to one another, as do players S2 and S4; each player serves, and that player's partner catches the ball after it has bounced and serves it back (figure 4.10). After a time the two players on each side of the net switch sides and do the same thing from their new position. This can also be done with only two players, serving diagonally to each other and occasionally switching which side they are serving from (playing in the positions of S1 and S3 from the diagram to start, then switching to positions S2 and S4).

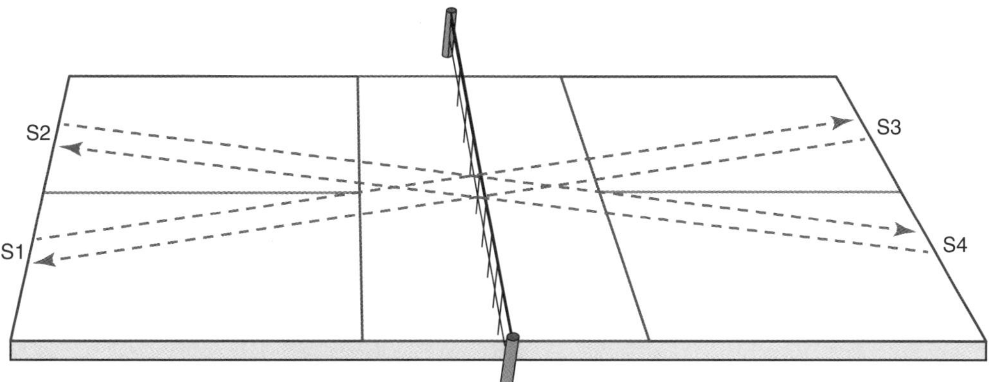

Figure 4.10 Serve and catch drill.

SERVE TO A TARGET

Using chalk, mark a target area on the court. Two players (S1 and S2) set up behind the baseline on the opposite side of the net with a supply of balls between them. Players S1 and S2 serve, aiming for the target area (figure 4.11). While serving deep to the backhand of your opponents is a critical skill to have in your arsenal, you can move the targets to different locations for practice.

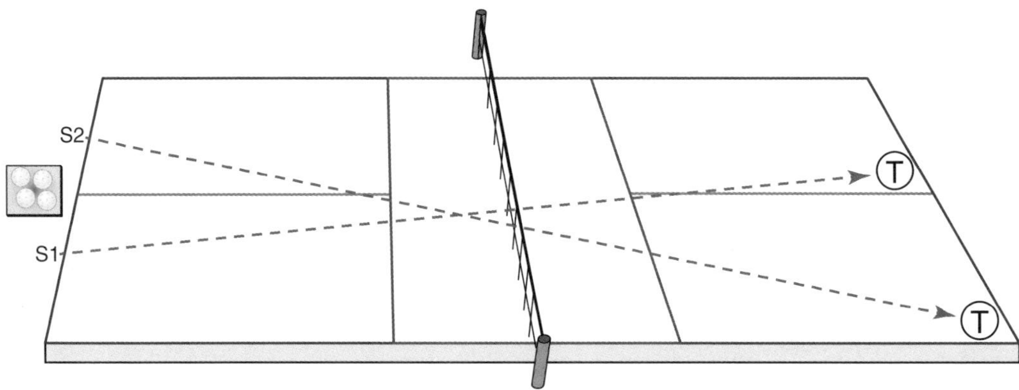

Figure 4.11 Serve to a target drill.

SERVE, RETURN, AND GO TO THE NET

This drill simulates the first part of a typical rally in pickleball. The server (S) serves crosscourt to the returner (R), who hits a slow, deep groundstroke to the backhand corner of the court directly across the net (figure 4.12). Immediately after the hit, following their own return forward and using the momentum of their swing, R moves quickly to the non-volley line. They should keep the paddle in front of them as they move forward and assume a ready position as soon as they reach the NVZ line.

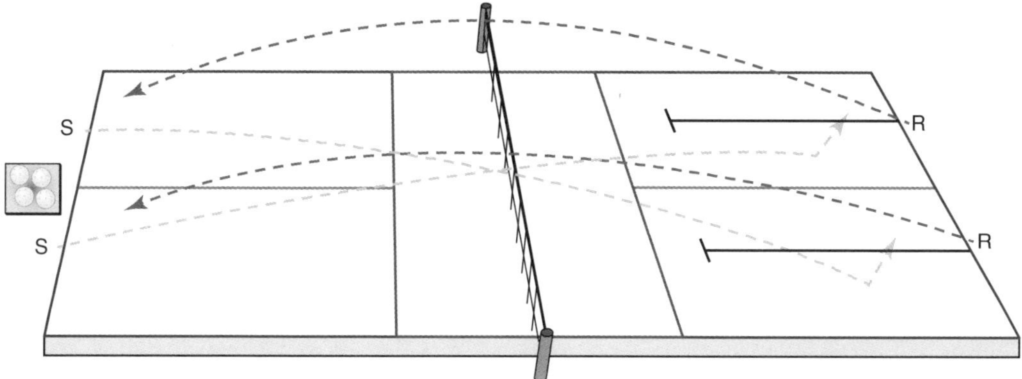

Figure 4.12 Serve, return, and go to the net drill.

Match Point

The serve and return of serve are the only two shots in a game of pickleball that cannot be returned without first allowing the ball to bounce. Because these are the two shots that begin every rally in a game, perfecting these two skills will bolster your confidence as the game continues. Every time you're on the pickleball court, concentrate on serving over the net and deep in the opponent's service court (perhaps adding the occasional short crosscourt serve) and returning every serve deep. You'll find that your pickleball game will improve by hitting these simple shots consistently to begin each rally!

CHAPTER

5

Volley

The volley in pickleball deserves special consideration because of the importance of the non-volley zone (NVZ) or "kitchen." It is a fault for any player hitting a volley to contact the NVZ during any part of their shot, including stepping into the NVZ due to any continuing momentum after their shot has been made.

A volley is any shot hit in the air before the ball bounces. A volley can be a soft shot like a dink or a hard drive struck with force from just outside the NVZ near the net. High-level play often sees a flurry of rapid volleys back and forth between players at the NVZ line, broken up by softer volleys (resets) aimed low toward the opponent's feet to stop the high-speed barrage.

Volleys are frequently used as a return of a ball that travels close to the top of the net and that is often driven with force. The ball coming your way may be a groundstroke, where the ball has already bounced before it is hit, or another volley. This volley is most often executed from a position just behind the NVZ, and it may be either offensive or defensive in nature. A volley can be more offensive if you make contact with the ball near or above the height of the net, because the flight path of the ball that you hit can be aimed downward, possibly with spin, allowing you to put more force on the ball and making the shot more difficult for your opponent to return. A volley is usually more defensive if you make contact with the ball below the height of the net, because the flight path of the ball that you hit is upward, giving your opponent the opportunity to return the ball with an aggressive rally-winning shot if your defensive volley is not soft enough to drop low into the NVZ, as with a dink (see chapter 6).

A defensive volley or reset is a good time to use a looser grip. This absorbs energy from the incoming shot, allowing for your soft placement of the ball low, near your opponent's' feet.

Defensive and offensive shots depend on a player's attitude. If a ball is hit as an easy pop-up high toward their forehand, a player looking for a chance to take the offensive advantage will be ready to hit this shot downward sharply, at the opponent's feet or out of their reach. A player not looking for this chance may lose the opportunity to end the rally and instead hit a return that allows their opponents to continue play. Similarly, an offense-minded player forced to hit a low defensive shot like a dink can still put pressure on their opponent by hitting the soft shot at their feet or low to the backhand, areas that many players find challenging.

Developing a strong net (NVZ) game, along with an attitude geared toward methodically creating and capitalizing on offensive opportunities, is crucial to your success as a pickleball player. The ability to volley with control, strength, and confidence is a crucial part of the successful net game.

You Can Do It

EXECUTING THE VOLLEY

When you are 8 or 9 feet (about 3 meters) from the net, you have far less time to react to a hard-driven ball coming at you than when you are 20 to 22 feet (about 7 meters) from the net for a forehand or backhand groundstroke. Therefore, being prepared both physically and mentally not only to stop the ball just after it crosses the net but also to return it aggressively may be a challenge that requires extra time and energy. From a balanced ready position (described in chapter 2), track the ball with your eyes as it leaves the opponent's paddle and approaches the net (figures 5.1 and 2*a*). As the ball comes toward you, move your body and paddle in line with it. Contact the ball above the height of the net in front of your body with a blocking motion (5.1 and 2*b*). Straighten the arm from the elbow and shoulder as contact is made. Think *block and push or punch*. With a firm grip on the paddle, use short, steady movements—no backswing, no wrist action, nothing jerky—and follow through slightly toward the target (5.1 and 2*c*). Remember that you cannot contact the NVZ while volleying your shot. Do not step forward into the NVZ during any part of your volley motion!

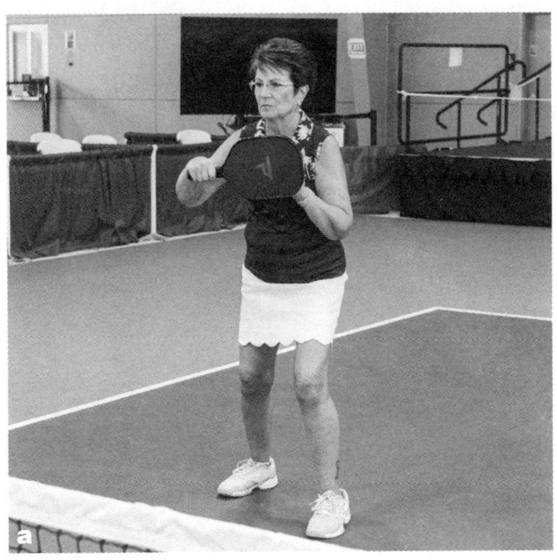

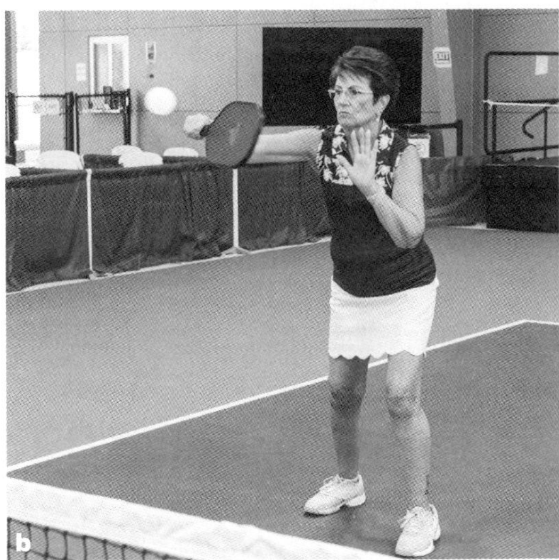

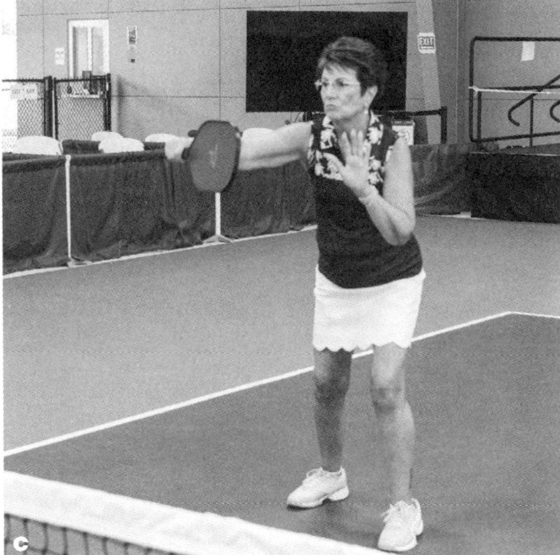

Figure 5.1 Block and push volley from backhand position: (*a*) preparation, (*b*) contact, and (*c*) follow-through.

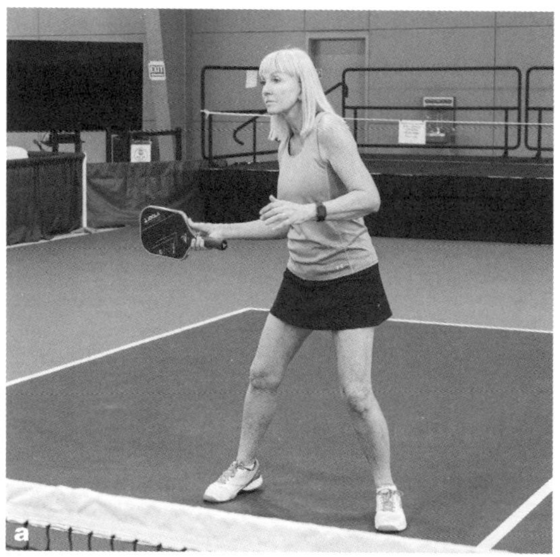

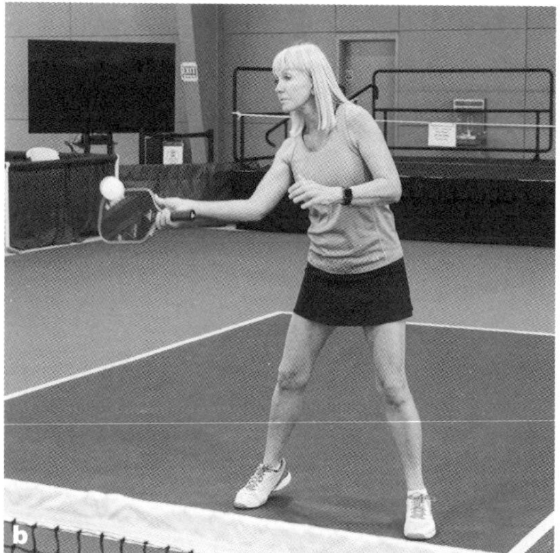

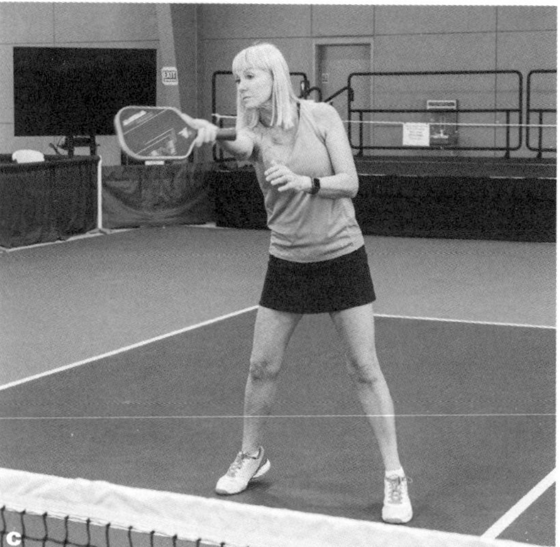

Figure 5.2 Block and push volley from forehand position: (*a*) preparation, (*b*) contact, and (*c*) follow-through.

Some advanced players use an alternative method when executing a volley. They apply force behind the volley by rotating the wrist when contacting the ball and not allowing the arm to straighten completely (figures 5.3 and 5.4). The follow-through when volleying with wrist action is more across the body rather than toward the net. The advantage of using this method of volleying is that it requires less time to return the

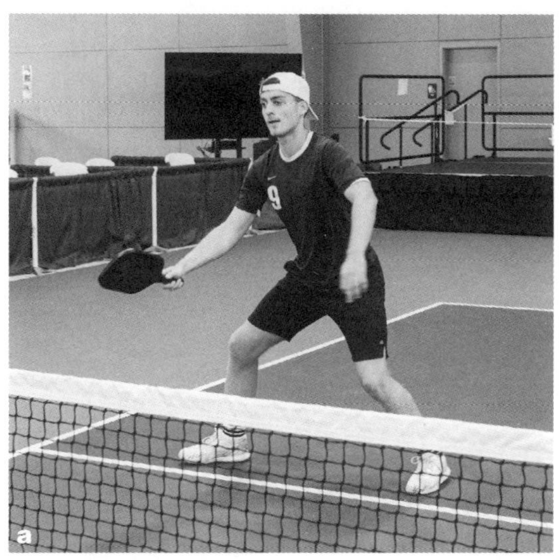

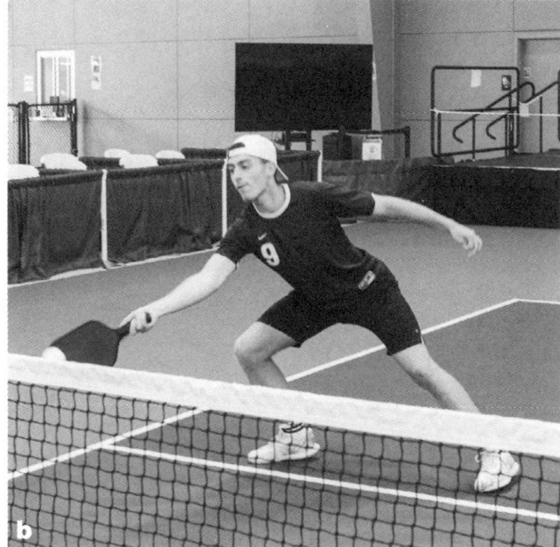

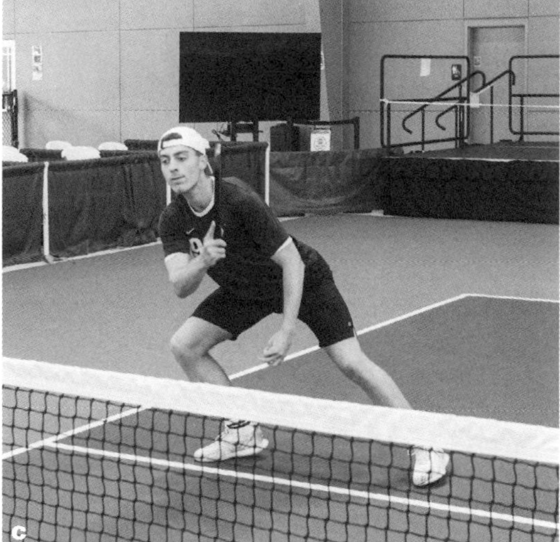

Figure 5.3 Forehand volley with wrist rotation: (*a*) preparation, (*b*) contact, and (*c*) follow-through.

paddle to a strong volley position in preparation for the next play. The ball should follow an up-to-down trajectory—up when you contact the ball and down as it crosses the net. Advanced players also add topspin to their volleys to exaggerate the ball's trajectory as it drops down over the net, keeping hard-hit shots lower, where they are more difficult to return, as well as in play, rather than sailing out of bounds as a ball without spin would be likely to end up.

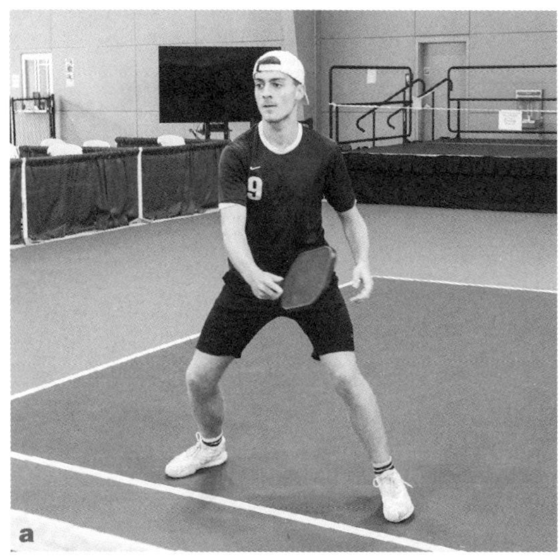

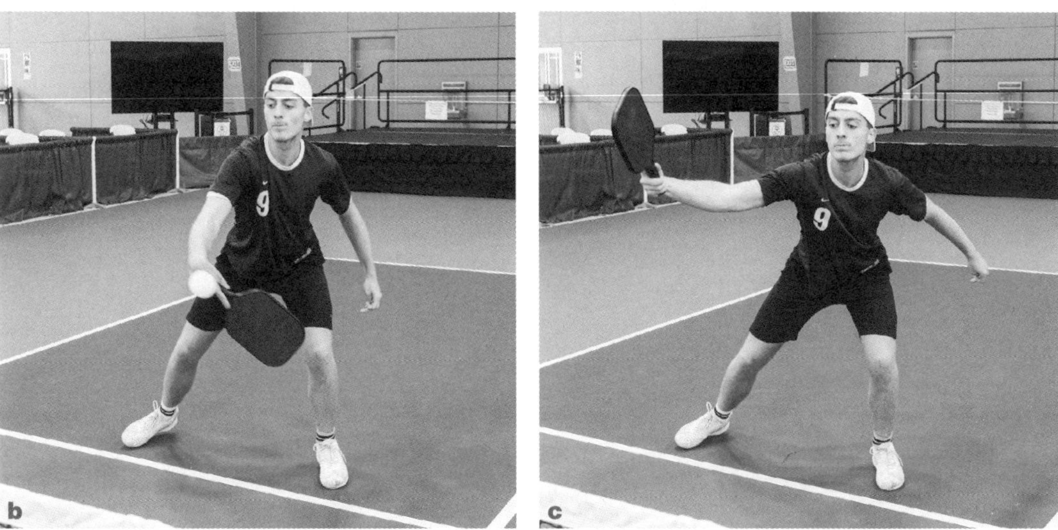

Figure 5.4 Backhand volley with wrist rotation: (*a*) preparation, (*b*) contact, and *(c)* follow-through.

There are many variations to executing these rapid volleys, especially as more players bring skills learned in other sports. Another technique for volleying that more advanced players use is to sweep the paddle across the front of the body while contacting the ball (figure 5.5). When you anticipate the ball coming toward your left shoulder, meet the ball with the face of the paddle and then cut across behind the ball with a sweeping motion of your paddle arm. The follow through is in front and

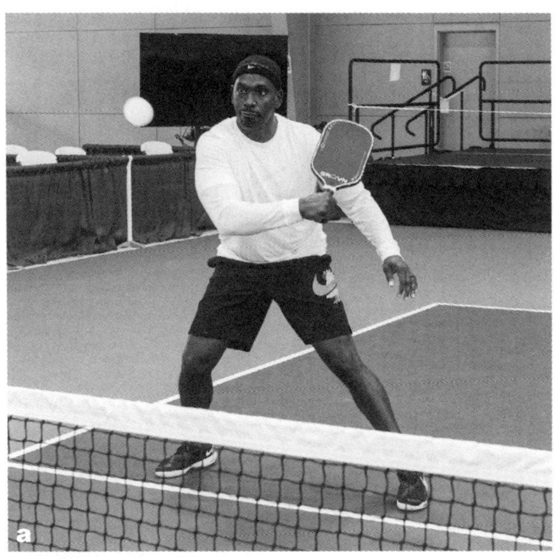

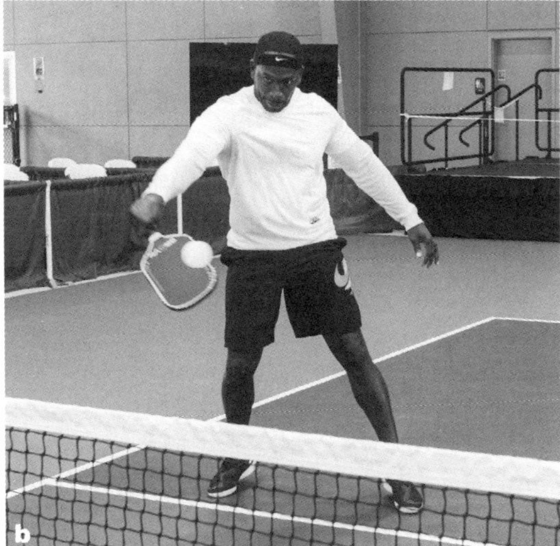

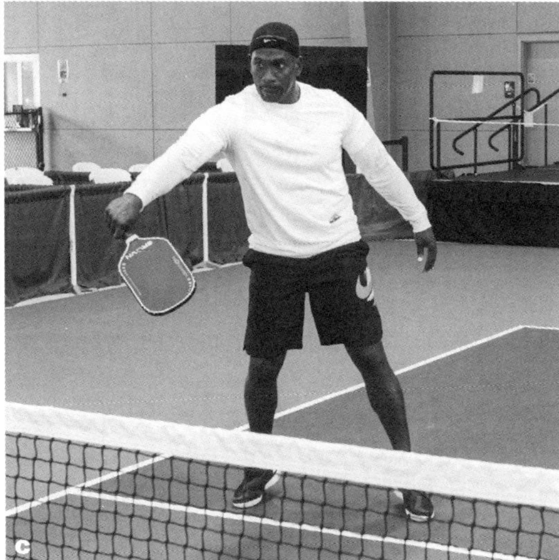

Figure 5.5 Backhand volley sweeping paddle across body: (*a*) preparation, (*b*) contact, and (*c*) follow-through.

to the right of your body. A sweeping volley is a challenging maneuver, so it requires a lot of practice.

Regardless of which method you use, you should make solid contact with the ball and then immediately prepare for another shot. The paddle and player should always return immediately to their ready position, with the paddle up and in front, prepared for the next quick volley coming their way. If that next shot coming toward them is a softer, slower ball, they have time to adjust. In contrast, if they are preparing for a slow shot, they will likely not have the reaction speed to handle an unexpected fast ball.

Your demeanor at the NVZ should be confident and strong. Let your attitude convey that you want the ball to come right at you because you're willing and able to return it! Face the net with flexed knees. Be light on your feet, ready to move. Hold the paddle up in front of you, and focus fully on the ball. While you are mentally and physically prepared to face a variety of attacking shots, you should also be alert to any hard-hit ball that is aimed too high. One of the easiest ways to win a rally is to simply allow your opponent's shot to go long or wide, out of bounds. Hitting a shot that would have been out does nothing but prolong a rally you should have already won and give your opponents another chance.

If you have time to direct your volley—and a strong, consistent "ready" position helps give you this time—send it down the middle between the opponents or to an open space. Volleying the ball right back at your opponent's feet, especially if the opponent is moving from deep in the court to the net, is often a good shot, encouraging them to hit a weak return. As always, if you have more time than just a reflexive effort to get the ball over the net, an offensive outlook will help you select a shot and target for your volley that helps your side gain an advantage and puts your opponent in a worse, more defensive position.

There will still also be times when your volley is a defensive move—you just want to keep the ball in play. A defensive volley can occur when you're at the net and the ball is hit so far to the side that you're unable to move your body behind it (figures 5.6 and 5.7). Therefore, you have to take a lunging step with the leg toward the oncoming ball and reach for it, hoping that the ball will rebound off of your paddle. If the ball is coming with force over the net and you're able to place your paddle in line with it, the ball will likely rebound off the paddle and go over the net. At least you've kept the ball in play! Do be aware, though, of where you are positioned on the court: if you are positioned correctly to cover the angles with your partner, most balls that you need to lunge for may be going out of bounds.

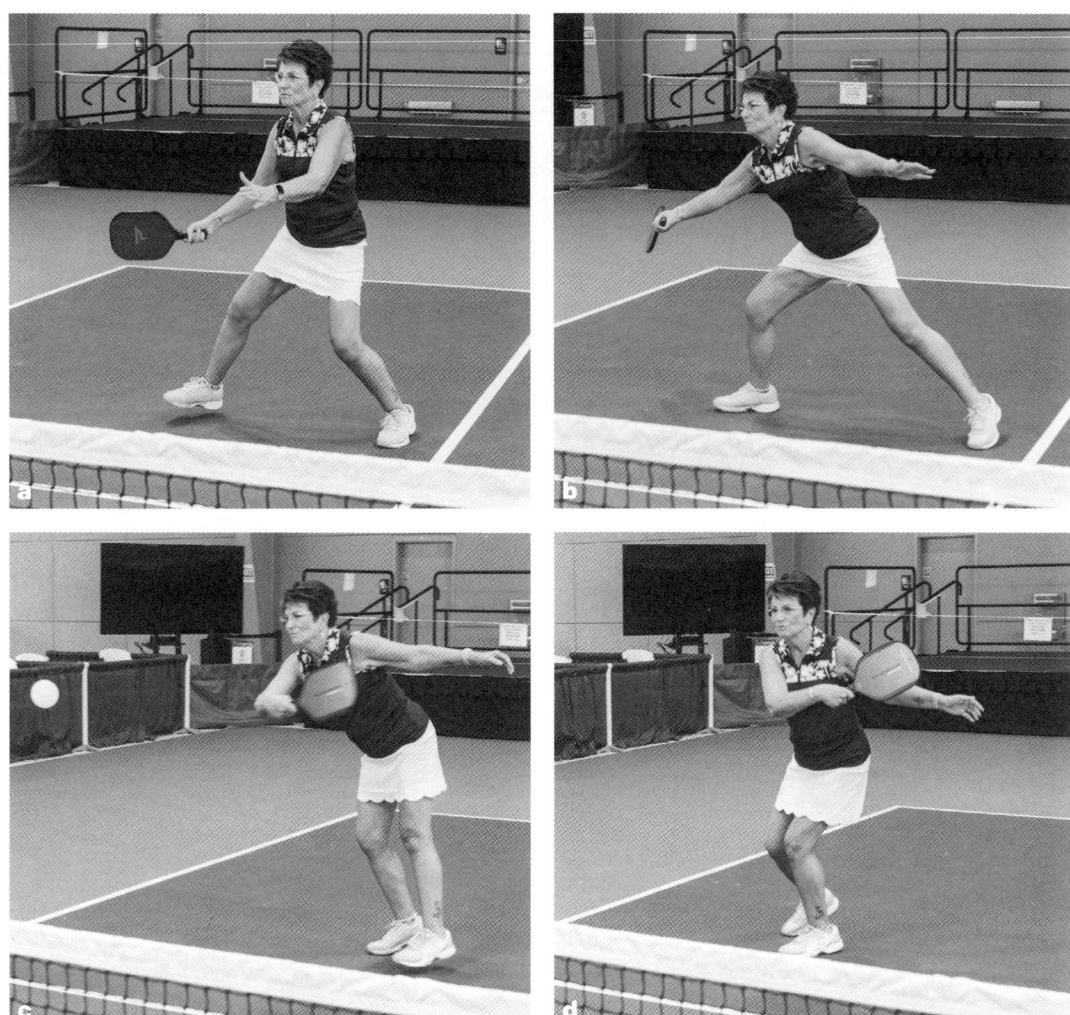

Figure 5.6 Executing a defensive volley to the right: (*a*) lunging toward the ball, (*b*) preparation, (*c*) contact, and (*d*) follow-through.

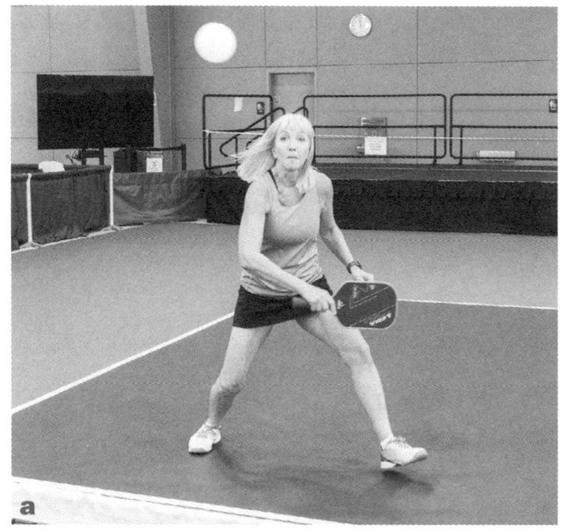

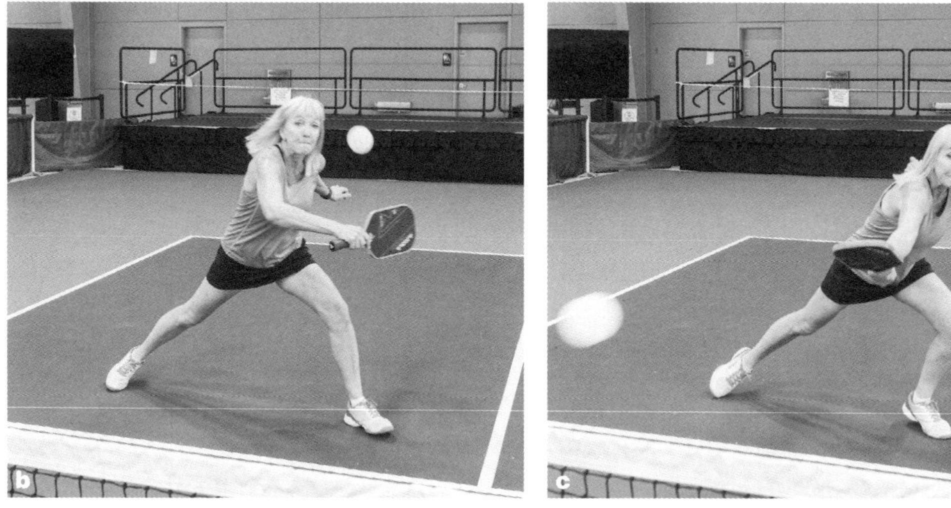

Figure 5.7 Executing a defensive volley to the left: (*a*) approach, (*b*) contact, and (*c*) follow-through.

While learning the volley, you need to fully understand the rules related to the non-volley zone (NVZ), mentioned earlier. The NVZ is the flat, two-dimensional area of the court bounded by the two sidelines, the non-volley line, and the net. The lines are considered to be part of the NVZ, but the air space above the NVZ can be entered with your paddle and body, such as during follow-through of a volley. Quite often, the paddle in a ready position will be above this area even before the swing and follow-through.

Volleying involves the swing, follow-through, and momentum from the action. If the paddle or any part of the player or anything the player is wearing touches the NVZ as you contact the ball or during the follow-through, it is a fault. Even after the player's volleying motion is over and the ball is dead, if the player's momentum carries them into the NVZ (including the lines), it is a fault. The most common NVZ fault is a foot fault with the player stepping forward as they complete their volley. If even the toe of one shoe contacts the NVZ—including the line—during any part of the volley or its momentum, it is a fault.

When moving from deep in the court to a position behind the NVZ, consider not going too close to the line. Stopping a few inches back from the line will enable you to take a short step forward without stepping into the NVZ while you are volleying. If the ball coming to you isn't coming with much force, you might have time to put more force into your return shot, which might result in taking a small step forward. Know your own game: if you tend to take this short forward step, leave yourself enough space to do that without committing a fault.

More to Choose and Use

HALF VOLLEY, OR SHORT HOP

As opposed to the volley, which is a shot taken when the ball is still in the air, before it has bounced, the "half volley" is hit immediately after the ball has bounced. The half-volleyer's paddle contacts the ball much lower than with a typical groundstroke. It is a reaction shot taken most often as you're approaching the net and the ball has been directed to your feet. You bend at the hips and knees and place the paddle just behind the bouncing ball, causing the ball to rebound back over the net. After ball contact, follow through, up and toward the net. You can execute the half volley from your forehand or your backhand side (figures 5.8 and 5.9). Your distance from the net determines how far open the

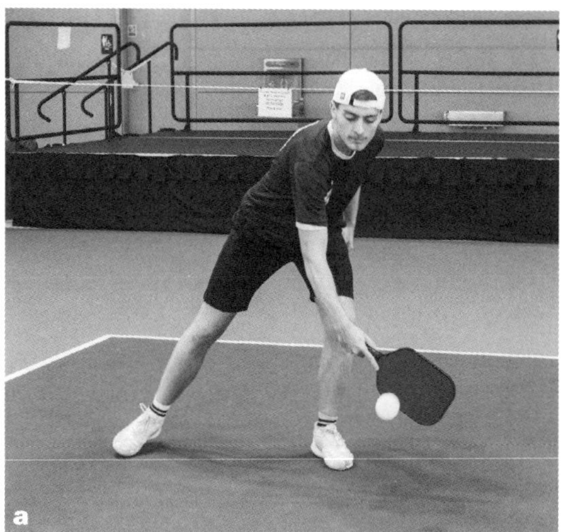

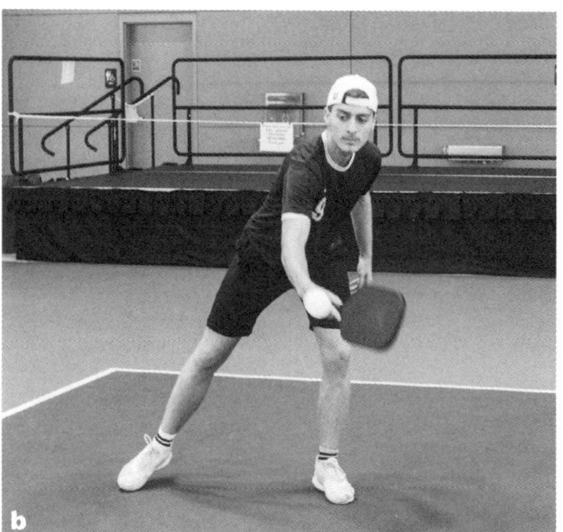

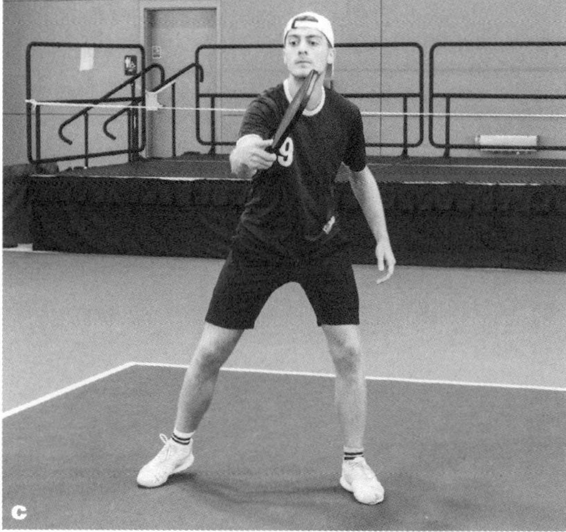

Figure 5.8 Hitting a backhand half volley (*a*) in position, (*b*) contact, and (*c*) follow-through.

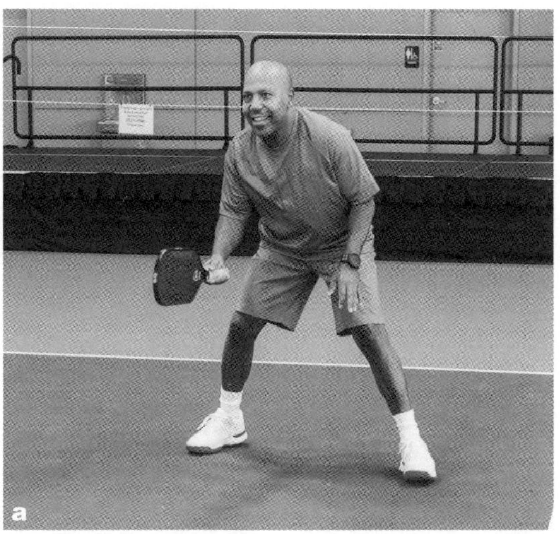

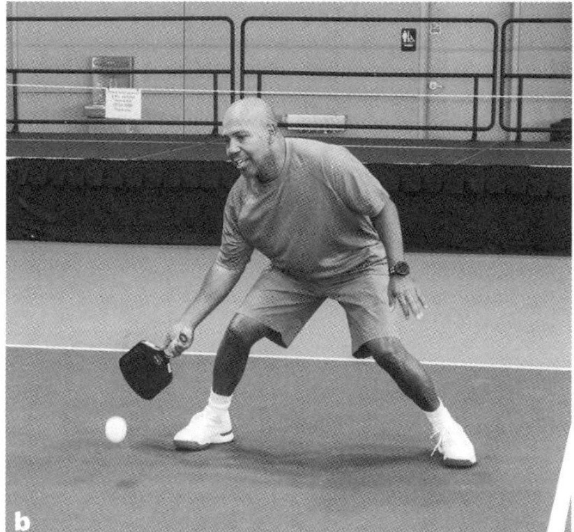

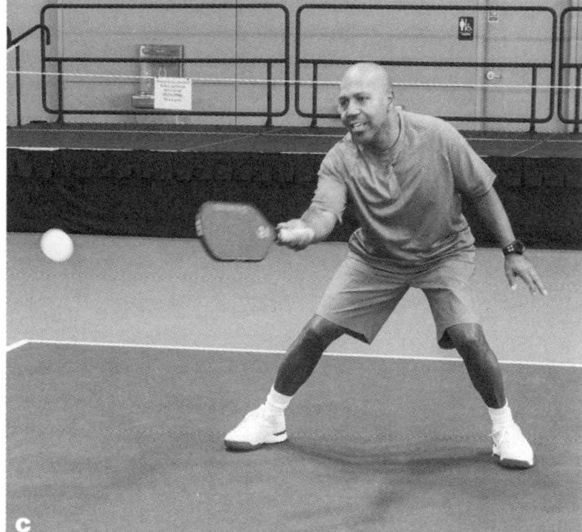

Figure 5.9 Hitting a forehand half volley (*a*) in position, (*b*) contact, and (*c*) follow-through.

face of the paddle must be for the ball to clear the net. The closer you are to the net, the more open the paddle face. Although a half volley is usually a defensive shot, it can sometimes become an offensive shot if it surprises an opponent who thought that the rally had already been won.

Note that "half volley" is a tennis term and misleading in pickleball. Per pickleball rules, the *half volley is not a volley at all* in terms of the NVZ. Since the ball has bounced before it is struck, there are no restrictions to entering the NVZ during or after this shot. For this reason, in pickleball, the term "short hop," borrowed from baseball, is less confusing than calling any non-volley a "half volley."

DROP VOLLEY

The drop volley can be a very effective shot when you are in a strong volleying position at the net and the opponent is deep in the court. Instead of executing a normal volley, loosen your grip slightly and give with the paddle, decreasing the force behind the hit. Stop the follow-through immediately after hitting the ball. The drop volley is a soft shot that

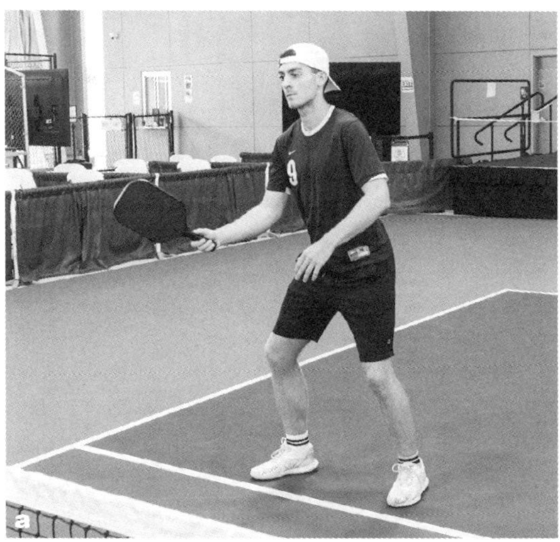
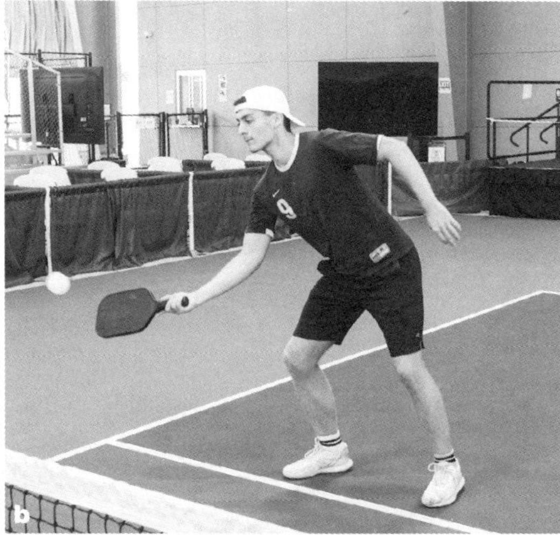
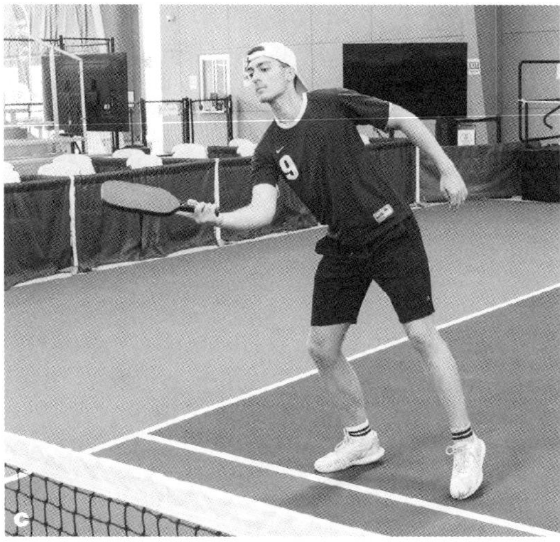
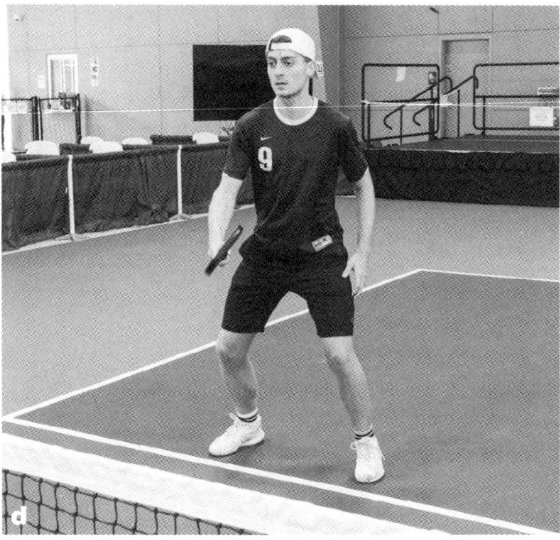

Figure 5.10 Executing a forehand drop volley (*a*) approach, (*b*) preparation, (*c*) contact, and (*d*) follow-through.

requires practice and finesse. Direct the shot to a shallow spot just inside one of the sidelines. The opponent, expecting a hard, deep volley, will have trouble getting to the ball, and if the opponent manages to return the shot, it will likely be a setup for you to put the ball away to win the rally. A drop volley can be done with the forehand (figure 5.10) or the backhand (figure 5.11). Adding some slice or backspin can cause the drop volley to bounce lower, making it even more difficult to return.

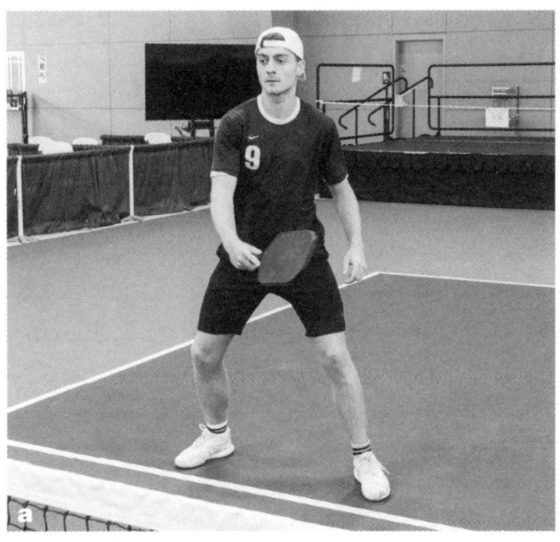

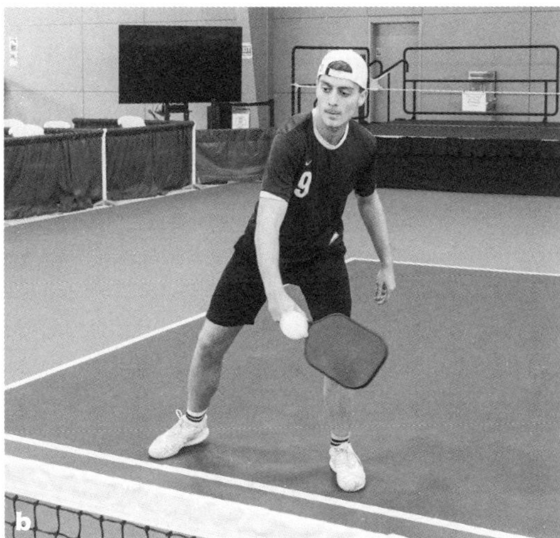

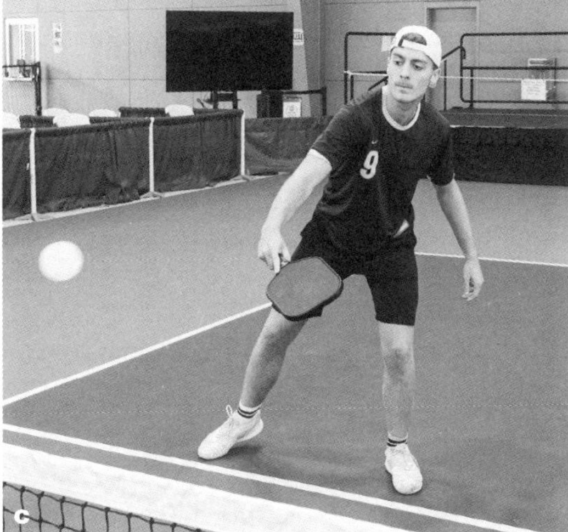

Figure 5.11 Executing a backhand drop volley (a) preparation, (b) contact, and (c) follow-through.

Take It to the Court

Recognizing errors that you commit and then being able to correct them will make you a better player. Here are some common errors and tips for correcting them.

Hitting the ball with little force and control

- *Concentrate on being ready.* Keep your body in a relaxed, balanced position, and hold the paddle roughly chest high between you and the net. As soon as you see the direction of the ball, move the paddle into a strong blocking position in line with the oncoming ball. Keep all the action in front of you where you can see it and control it.
- *Focus on going to the ball rather than letting the ball come to you and getting your paddle into position quickly.* Contacting the ball after it has passed the line of your shoulders means that you're late in attempting to execute the volley.

Hitting the ball into the net

- *Be patient—don't rush your shot.* See the ball actually hit the paddle, and consciously direct your follow-through to a specific, advantageous area of the opponent's court.
- *Focus on the face of the paddle being square to the net.* If it is in a closed position, the ball will travel in a downward direction off of the paddle.
- *Grip the paddle firmly at the moment of contact with the ball.* A loose grip will cause you to lose control of the paddle and decrease the force applied to the hit.
- *See the ball contact the sweet spot on the face of the paddle.* Strive for consistency in the force of your hit.

Hitting the ball too long

- *Concentrate on squaring the face of the paddle.* If the ball is coming to you high, punch or swing downward at the ball; if the ball is closer to the top of the net, square it.
- *Think of pushing or punching the ball back and downward over the net.* Keep your arm movements short, controlled, and from the shoulder.

Hitting the ball out of bounds to either side

- *Strive to place the hit down the middle.* Trying to be too perfect in your hit can cause it to be erratic. Keep your movements simple and controlled and your blocking paddle face roughly parallel to the net.

Give It a Go

Volleying well is a key part of becoming a well-rounded pickleball player. The time spent in practicing the skills required for a good net game will have a strong impact on your overall success on the court.

GROUNDSTROKE AND VOLLEY

One player (P) stands at a baseline. The other player (called V, since they will be hitting the volleys) sets up near the NVZ on the opposite side of the net. P bounces the ball and hits it with moderate force directly across the net to V, who volleys it (before it bounces) back to P. They keep the rally going as long as possible, with P hitting groundstrokes and V hitting volleys. V can also move closer to the NVZ as they get comfortable with their volleys, more closely simulating actual game play. Note: V should stay aware and avoid stepping into the NVZ. This drill can be done with 4 players on one court (2 Ps and 2 Vs) with rallies going on both left and right sides of the court (figure 5.12).

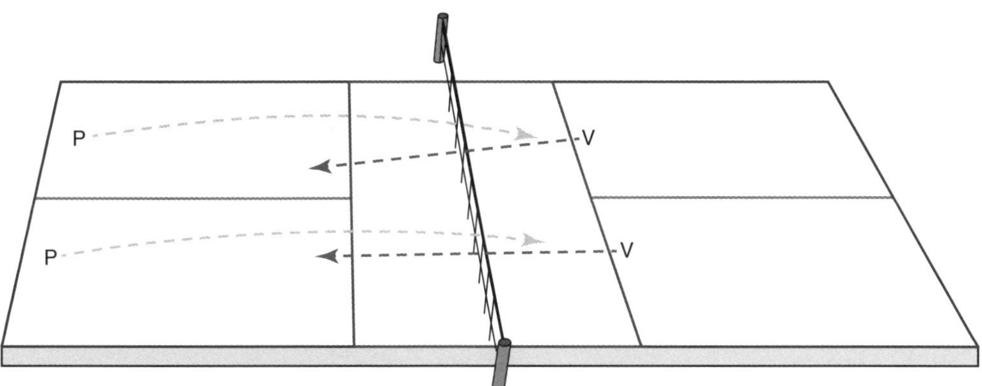

Figure 5.12 Groundstroke and volley drill.

VOLLEY OVER AND BACK

Four players take the court, one in each quadrant, just behind the NVZ. Each player volleys with the player directly across the net, sending the ball back and forth and attempting to keep the rally going for as long as possible (figure 5.13). Players can experiment with how hard these volleys are hit. It can be a great confidence booster to successfully complete a prolonged back-and-forth drill with your practice partner. Another variation is to step inside the NVZ so that you and your practice partner are about 10 feet (3 meters) apart, each a couple feet (roughly 60 cm) inside the zone. After volleying back and forth at this short range, when you step back out of the NVZ, it will feel like you have much more reaction time.

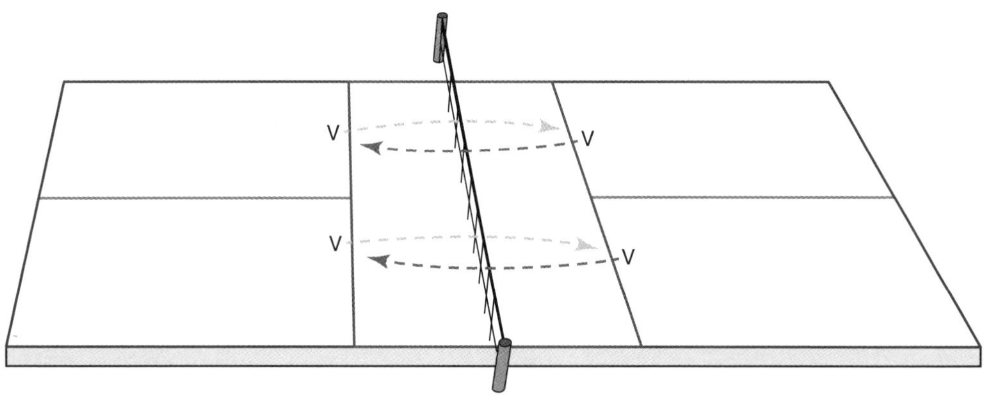

Figure 5.13 Volley over and back drill.

VOLLEY OVER AND BACK WITH FOOT-WORK

This is a variation of the Volley Over and Back drill. Two players take the court, standing directly opposite each other and just behind the NVZ line, near one sideline (figure 5.14). With each successful volley hit, they both take a sideways step with each foot. Another volley, another sideways movement. They should maintain their ready positions, moving together about half their shoulder width each time. The players should strive to stay directly opposite one another with a goal of successfully hitting volleys as they travel to the other side line. At that point they reverse directions and return to the starting sideline, again performing the footwork.

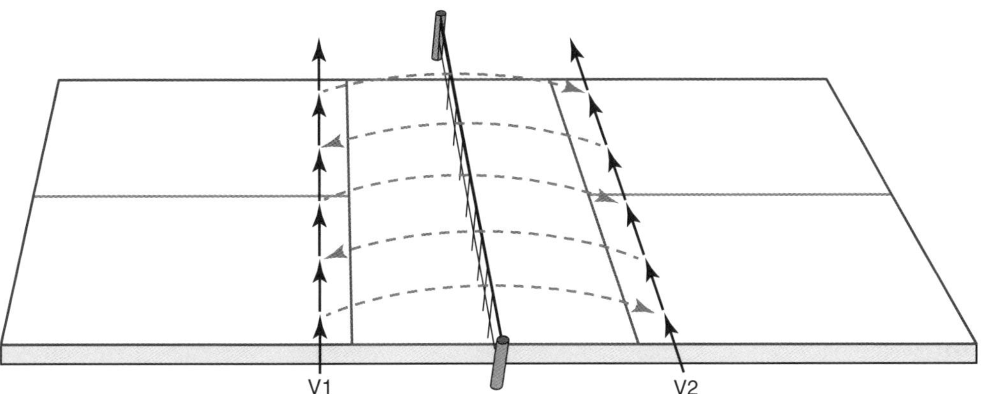

Figure 5.14 Volley over and back with footwork drill.

THROW AND HALF VOLLEY

F1 and F2 throw balls at the feet of HV1 and HV2, who are positioned in midcourt. HV1 and HV2 execute a half volley (figure 5.15). Alternatively, HV1 and HV2 can begin from behind the baseline and move into position to execute a half volley. After a few hits, the groups rotate. This can also be done with one F and one HV.

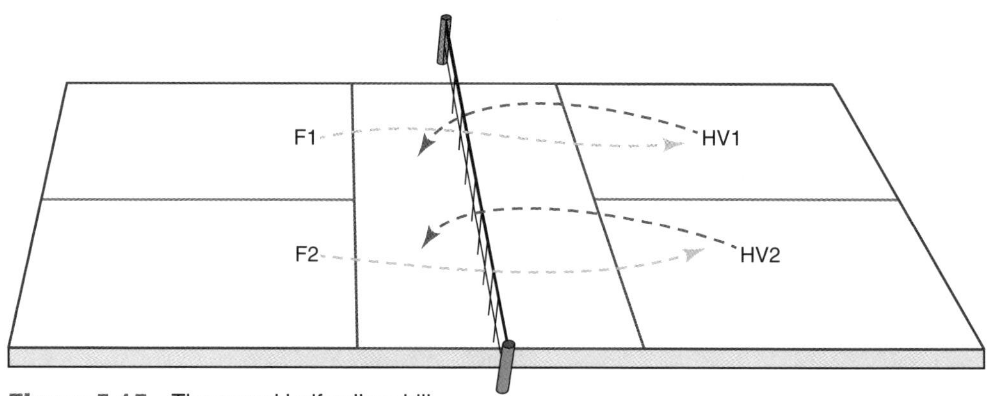

Figure 5.15 Throw and half volley drill.

Match Point

It is crucial to a player's success in a game of pickleball that they become comfortable playing at the net (really the NVZ). Being able to both execute a consistent and aggressive volley at the net and handle a rapid volley coming your way can make the difference between just being able to play the game and being able to play the game well. Be patient and persistent in learning how and when to volley and your game will improve tremendously.

CHAPTER

6

Dink

Over the years, the game of pickleball has changed from one dominated by forceful groundstrokes hit by players who were largely content to hit the ball hard from deep in their court to one dominated by a net game of soft, finessed shots hit by players waiting to pounce with a kill shot if the ball was hit too high, and now to a well-rounded game where competitive players must effectively use it all: soft, finessed shots and hard attacking drives both, along with skillful resets and varying spin and pace, to succeed at a high level.

The changing nature of the game has led to complaints that those who drive the ball hard on most shots—called "bangers"—aren't playing properly and should use more soft shots and finesse, even if they are winning their games. In fact, whatever works, safely and within the rules, is the right way to play competitively. Other players love nothing better than dinking back and forth, celebrating a long rally, laughing while getting exercise with friends. They might not even keep score. Their "right way" may be very different from the tournament player.

Although it is true that to be a good pickleball player you must learn and master several skills, none is more important—or more unique to pickleball—than the soft, low, controlled dink. The dink, executed from inside or near the non-volley zone (NVZ), may be hit either before or after the ball bounces with the intent of dropping the ball softly over the net to land in the opposing NVZ or near the opponent's feet. This forces them to hit their next shot upward, from a position that makes it very difficult to attack offensively. Your soft net game depends on your ability to execute consecutive dinks with success, from both the forehand and backhand sides.

Crucial to dinking and the soft game is comprehending the official rules pertaining to the NVZ. Imprint this in flashing bold letters in your mind forever: *If the ball bounces, you can go anywhere on your side of the court to return it!* When you are in this zone—7 feet (2.1 m) from the net and 20 feet (6.1 m) wide including the bounding sidelines and NVZ line—you cannot hit the ball before it bounces; if you do, it is a fault because it is a volley hit while in the NVZ. But *if* it bounces, you can be all the way to the net and hit the ball, providing you do not touch the net with any part of your body, clothing, or paddle. You also do not need to wait for the ball to bounce before entering the NVZ. As long as you do not volley the ball, allowing it to bounce before hitting it, you can be in this zone whenever you like.

You Can Do It

EXECUTING THE DINK

You and your partner stand just behind the NVZ line in a good ready position—well balanced, with your body weight over your feet and the knees slightly bent. Hold the paddle in front of your body at chest level. The head of the paddle is perpendicular to the ground in a position that allows for a quick, smooth movement to either side. You feel light on your feet, ready for the ball to come to you. If your opponent's return shot drops just over the net on your side, this scenario calls for a dink.

Move to the bouncing ball using measured steps, beginning to move as soon as you can see where the ball is going. Because you are no more than about 8 feet (2.4 m) from the net to start with, you don't have to travel very far to reach the ball. Finish your movement in a balanced position, feet planted wider than shoulders, with your paddle coming back for your shot and your knees and hips bent, placing you low to the ground (figure 6.1*a*). Reach for the ball with an open paddle face (6.1*b*) and contact the ball low to the ground with a lifting action (6.1*c*), trying to keep the ball in contact with the face of the paddle as long as possible (6.1*d*). Think *lift* rather than *hit*: a soft stroke much like the motion of tossing a ball to a child who is just learning to catch.

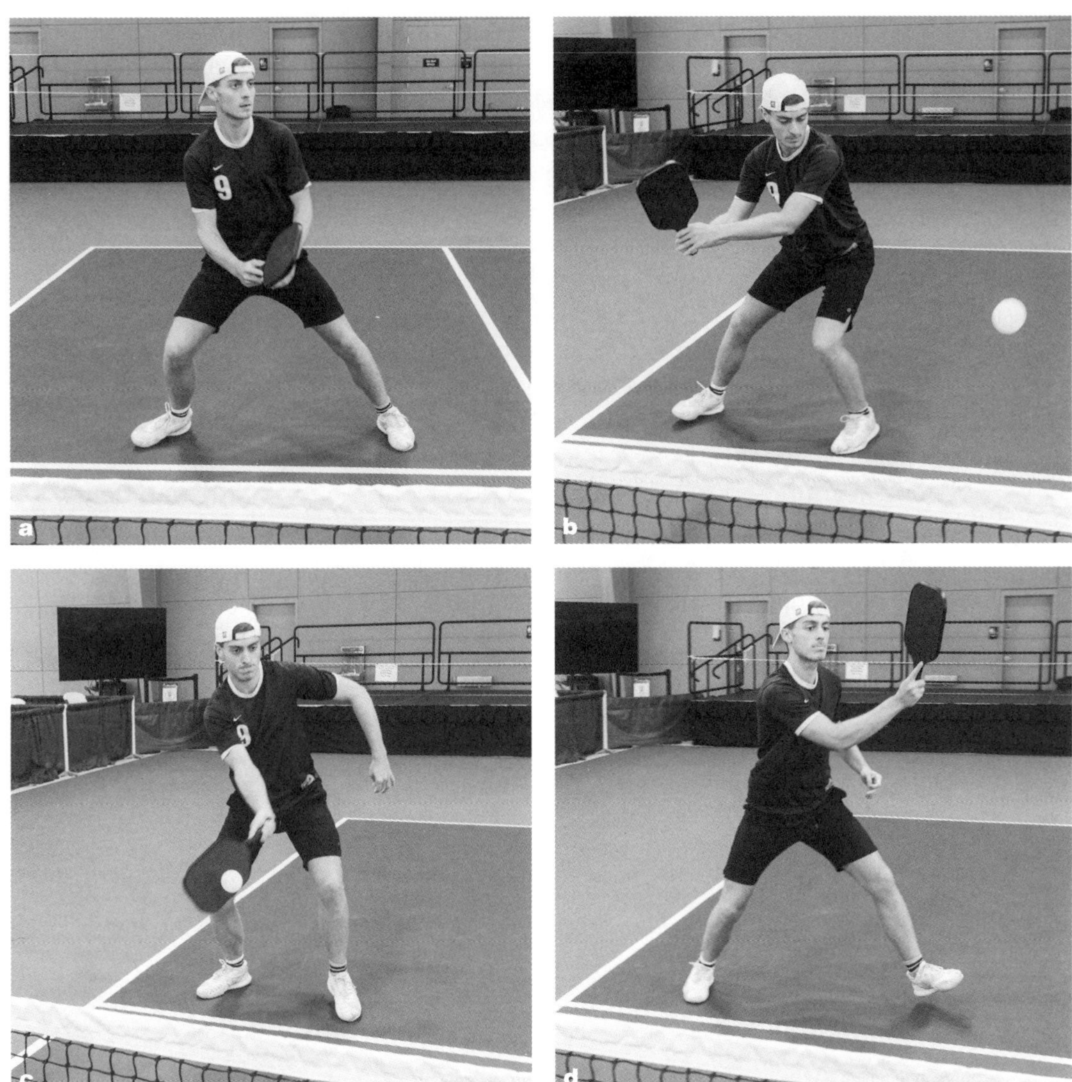

Figure 6.1 Executing a soft dink shot: (*a*) approach and position, (*b*) reach for the ball, (*c*) contact, and (*d*) follow-through.

The goal of your dink should be for the ball to arc softly over the top of the net and land in the NVZ close to the opponent's feet or another position that makes their return challenging and defensive. A dink should be a soft, controlled hit, well supported by a comfortable stance, with the impetus of the hit coming from your arm, which should move from the shoulder with no wrist or elbow action, much like a pendulum. Think of the paddle as an extension of your arm.

The result of a good dink should be an attempted dink coming from the other side of the net (figure 6.2). Your target can be straight across the net or crosscourt. A well-hit crosscourt dink will force one member of the opposing team to leave their area of the court to make the return shot, which creates an opening in their defensive positioning and may set up a put-away shot by you or your partner.

When executing any shot intended to just clear the top of the net, bear in mind that the height of the net in the center of the court is 2 inches (about 5 cm) shorter than the height of the net over the sidelines—34 inches (86 cm) high in the center as opposed to 36 inches (90 cm) high at the sideline. This means that any shot of yours traveling over the net in the center of the court is a higher-percentage shot.

Diagonal shots, or cross-court shots, by their nature tend to take advantage of this by passing over the midsection of net.

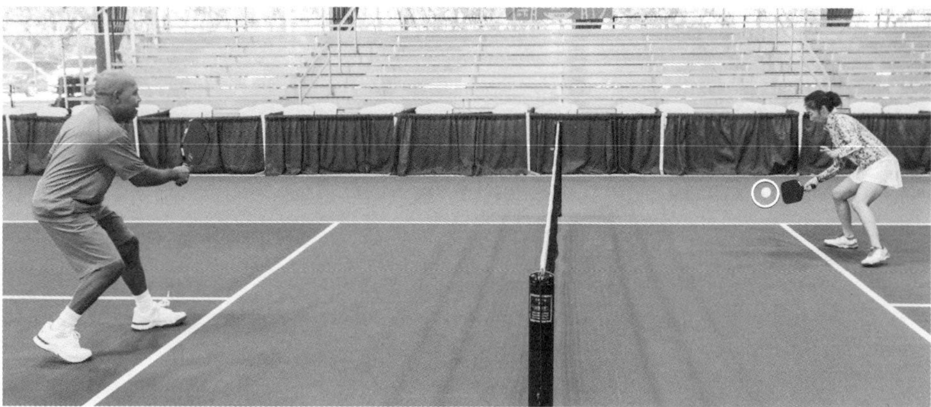

Figure 6.2 Dink returned with another dink.

More to Choose and Use

USING THE DINK IN GAME PLAY

In the "total doubles" game, a player and a partner stand behind their baseline. The ball travels over the net and lands deep in the service court diagonally across from the server. One player on the receiving team is positioned deep to return the serve, and the other stands behind the NVZ line (figure 6.3*a*). Immediately after the serve is returned, the receiver begins to advance forward to a position side by side with the partner (6.3*b*). The rate of advancement is based on the mobility and speed of each returner, with the focus being on balanced movement toward the NVZ. Once both players are positioned at the NVS, the receiving team is in a strong offensive position at the net and the serving team is deep in their court waiting for the ball to bounce before they can return it (6.3*c*).

The serving team's goal is to return the ball with one of the various shots (a drop, a drive, or a lob, for example) that allows them the opportunity to follow up their shot to the net. Assuming they are successful, both teams are in position at the net to either volley or dink the ball (6.3*d*).

A rally continues until one team has committed a fault, usually by hitting their shot short (into the net) or out of bounds (either too long or too wide), landing outside the court boundary. This fault may happen when one team gains an advantage and is able to put the ball away by hitting it angled down with force, out of the opponent's reach, or by a player trying to keep a dink too low and hitting it into the net. Other common faults are entering the NVZ on a volley, allowing the ball to contact your body or non-paddle hand, or letting the ball bounce twice before it is hit. Depending on which team won the rally and which player—first or second server—was serving, it's a point, second serve, or side out (meaning that the ball goes to the opposing team for their first serve).

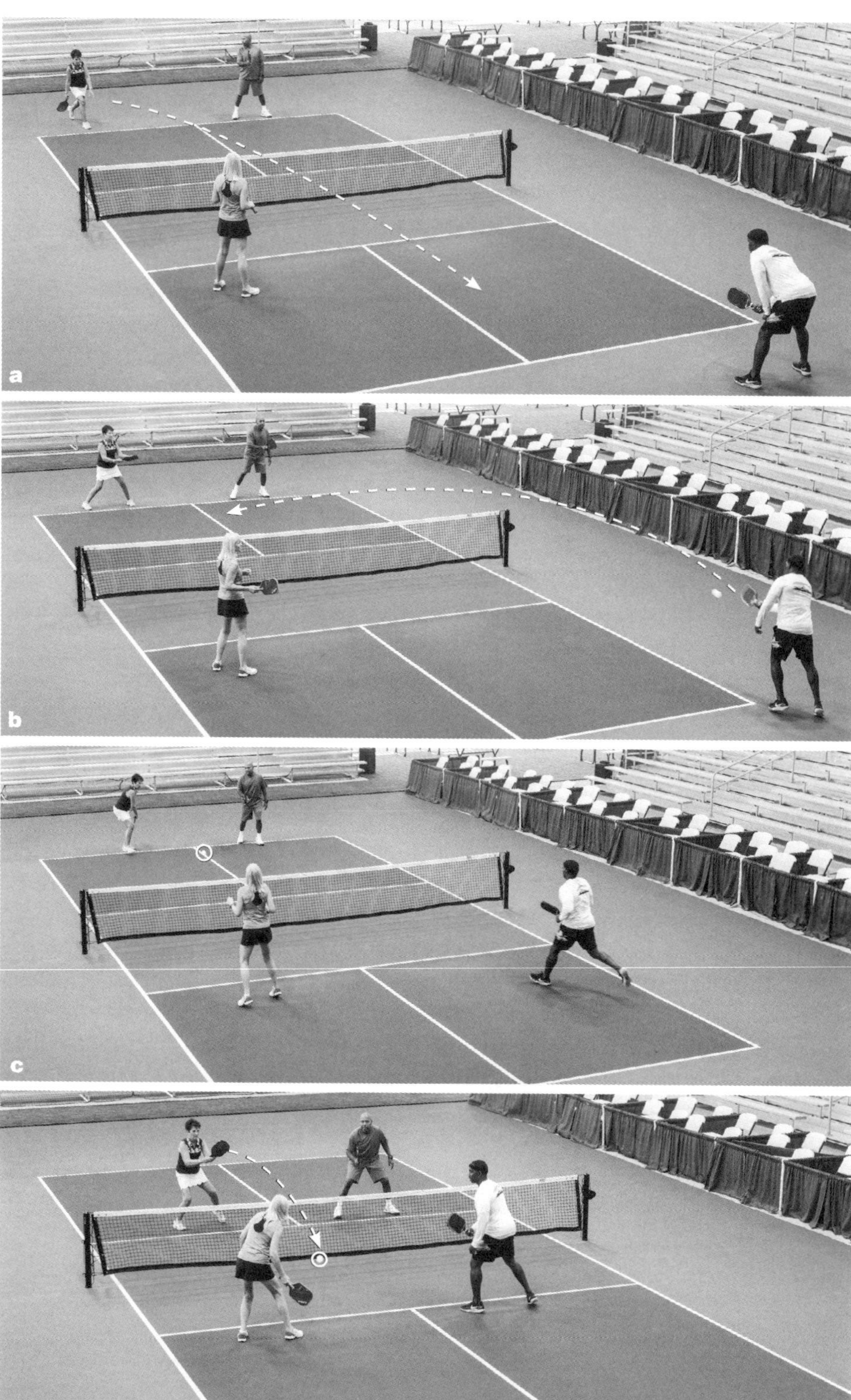

Figure 6.3 The shot sequence that places both teams in position to dink: (*a*) ball is served, (*b*) player returns the serve and begins approach to the NVZ line, (*c*) the server or the server's partner hits a drop shot and they begin approaching the NVZ line, and (*d*) all four players dinking at the net.

Take It to the Court

The success of your pickleball game is directly related to your success in dinking the ball. The following information should help you in correcting any errors that you might be committing.

The dink goes into the net

- *Focus on placing the face of the paddle underneath the ball as well as behind it.*
- *Make sure the face of the paddle is open as you contact the ball and use an upward motion.*
- *Watch the ball actually hit the sweet spot of the paddle.*
- *The arm should move forward and upward to help the ball clear the net. Try not to just make a short bunt or tap of the ball.*

The dink is hit too deep and too high

- *Think of lifting the ball, not hitting the ball.* The action involves the arm in a smooth, stroking motion pivoting at the shoulder like a pendulum. There is no backswing and only a short upward follow-through. If the ball goes too deep and high, you're probably swinging at it rather than lifting it with a soft touch.
- *Loosen your grip slightly (imagine a grip of 4, with 10 being the tightest) at the point of contact to soften the hit.*
- *Consider squaring the paddle face more.*
- *Be in a balanced position when you dink the ball.* If a short shot bounces before you hit it, you can move into the NVZ early so as to be in a comfortable ready position before your dink.

Missing to either the right or the left

- *Strive to hit the ball smoothly, in a soft arc, following a diagonal across the court where the net is lowest rather than straight toward the opponent directly opposite you. This path gives you more chances for a successful dink.* Avoid trying to be too perfect, aiming for the sidelines or directly over the net's highest points!
- *Maintain a balanced position behind the ball, moving into position early, as soon as you see the ball's path toward your side.*
- *Emphasize a deliberate extension of the paddle towards the target area.*

Give It a Go

The dink requires a soft, delicate touch. It's particularly challenging for players to learn how to shift between hitting a moving ball hard on one shot and then immediately applying finesse to a soft shot. Being able to feel the difference between a hard hit and a soft shot and execute them repeatedly back to back takes a great deal of time and practice even for players who have participated in other sports. During each of these drills, focus on the physical sensation—in your muscles and joints, in the shift of your body weight, in the impact of the ball on the paddle—of hitting a soft, delicate shot as opposed to a hard, forceful one. Eventually, your muscles will learn to respond to these varying shots with little or no conscious thinking required. Until then, practice.

DINK ACROSS

If there are four players, they should set up on the court with one in each quadrant, just outside the NVZ. If there are only two players in the drill, they should start directly across the net from each other. Each player pairs up with the player directly across the net, and each pair has a ball. One player per pair dinks the ball to the player across the net, who dinks it back. They keep the rally going as long as possible (figure 6.4). After several successful rallies, four players will dink the ball crosscourt, but if there are only two players, one slides over to be crosscourt from the other. Concentrate on executing the dink correctly and keeping the rally going.

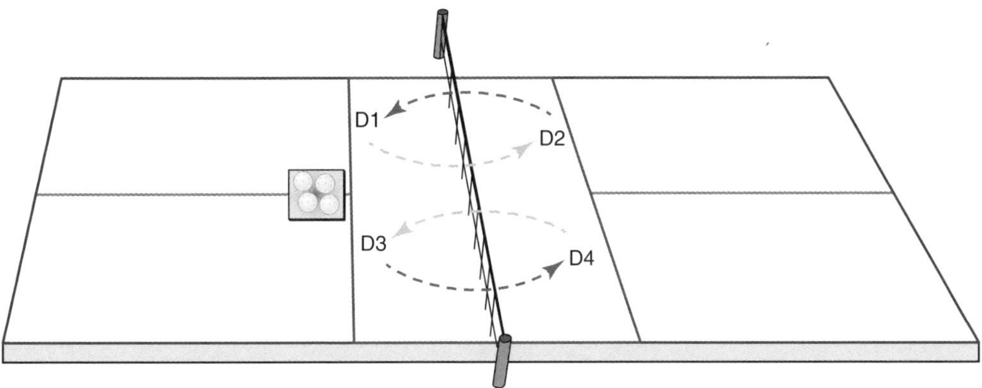

Figure 6.4 Dink across.

DINK GAME

Play a regular four-person game but keep the ball inside the NVZ using only the dink, either volleying or taking the shot after it bounces. If the ball goes into the net or lands beyond the NVZ line, it is a fault (figure 6.5). As it is also a fault to enter the NVZ while executing a volley, this is good practice for deciding when to allow the ball to bounce before hitting it and choosing the appropriate footwork to avoid a NVZ fault. If time allows, use regular scoring; a game is over when one team has scored 11 points. This game can be played as "singles" with just two players, using two of the four NVZ quadrants, either straight across the net from each other or crosscourt, on the diagonals.

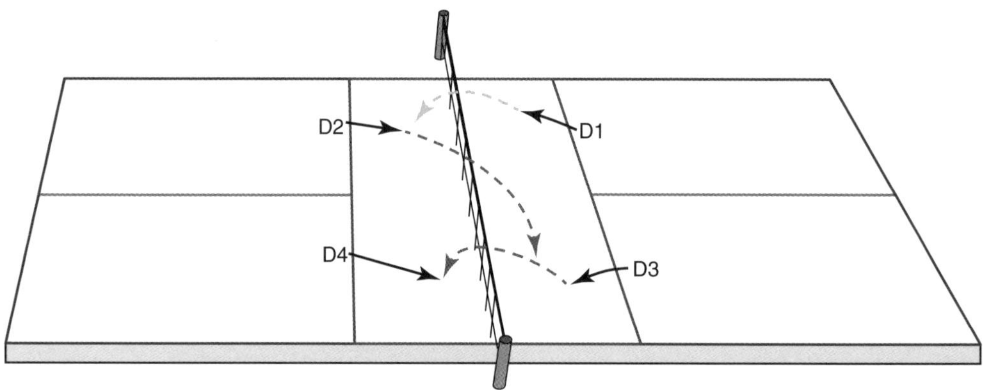

Figure 6.5 Dink game.

ANYTHING GOES

Four players—two on each side of the net—dink the ball back and forth, concentrating on moving the ball around and forcing footwork adjustments from the opposing players. Players call out the number of dinks. Immediately after "8" is called out, anything goes, meaning that any shot can be used anywhere in the court—you no longer utilize only dinks. It becomes a regular game using the entire court, but all players are already at the NVZ. When the rally ends, the players start again at the net, dinking and calling out the number of dinks.

Match Point

Being skilled at net play (in or near the NVZ) is very important to becoming a good pickleball player. The dink, executed with a soft touch and finesse, is a shot that might not be a frequent point winner by itself, but it will help prevent an effective attacking shot by your opponent, prolonging the rally. A well-placed offensive dink (as an example, one landing near the opponent's backhand foot) can encourage the opponent to make an error, committing a fault or hitting the ball too high, which will be a setup for an aggressive point-winning shot. The soft touch required to execute an effective dink requires a lot of practice and self-control, but the reward on the court is great.

CHAPTER

7

Lob

The lob is a lofted shot usually hit off a bounce that can be either offensive or defensive in nature. The object of lobbing is to take your opponents out of their preferred game, to force them away from a strong position at the non-volley line, making them move back in their court by hitting the ball in a high arc over their heads. A well-executed lob requires a feel for knowing how hard to hit the ball and how much loft to apply so that the ball clears the outstretched arm and paddle of the opponent but still lands inside the boundary lines.

You Can Do It

EXECUTING THE LOB

When executing a lob, approach the ball as if you were going to hit it with a groundstroke, dink, or other shot. The lob works best if it is unexpected. As you're tracking the ball with your eyes, move to the approaching ball using controlled, balanced steps. You should finish with your body partially facing the net and the sideline, with the bouncing ball between you and the net and to your right side (for the right-handed player). Once you are in a forward-stride position (facing the net with your left foot in front of the right one and your feet a comfortable distance apart) with the bouncing ball between you and the net and the ball lined up off of your front knee, open the face of the paddle and drop your paddle arm back and toward the ground (figure 7.1*a*-*b*). Swing your paddle arm forward and contact the ball with a lifting action, trying to keep the ball in contact with the face of the paddle for as long as possible as you shift your weight from your rear foot to your forward foot (7.1*c*). The forward swing of the paddle arm should move toward the target. Most important when executing a lob is to think of it as being a *soft lift* of the ball, not a brisk hit (7.1*d*).

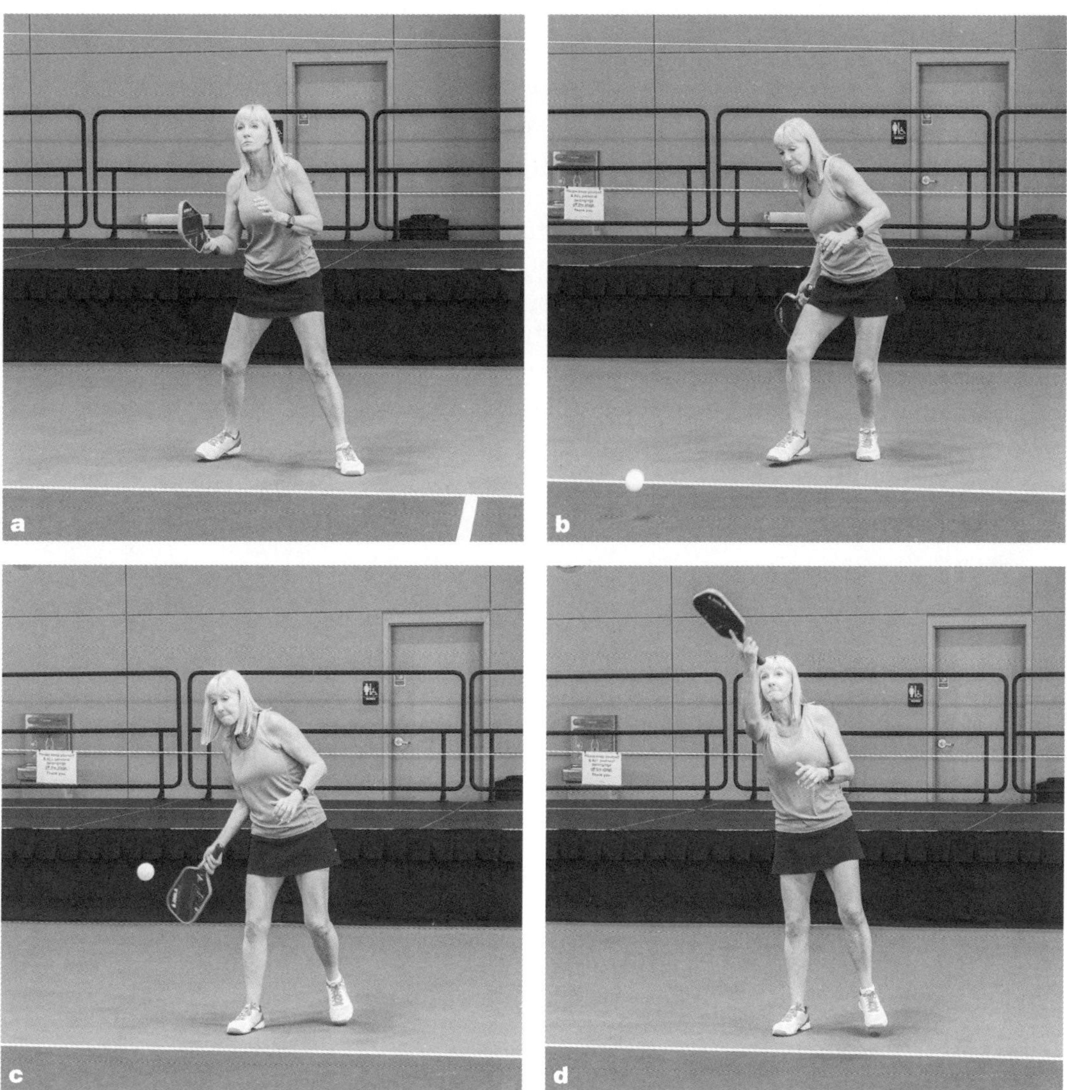

Figure 7.1 Executing the lob: (*a*) preparation, (*b*) backswing, (*c*) contact, and (*d*) follow-through.

Defensive Lob

You can use a defensive lob whenever you need time to recover from a desperate return of a well-placed shot from your opponents (figure 7.2*a* and *b*). You would use this type of shot if you are able to get your paddle on the ball, but the best you can do is to lob it deep in the opposing court to give you and your partner time to get back into position for the next shot. Hitting the ball with a high loft can allow your team a valuable extra couple seconds to reset. Often when hitting a defensive lob, you aren't in a position that is balanced enough to direct it. Under these circumstances, you should consider it a successful shot if you hit it over the heads of your opponents so that the ball lands inside the court or forces an awkward overhead return rather than a well-placed slam.

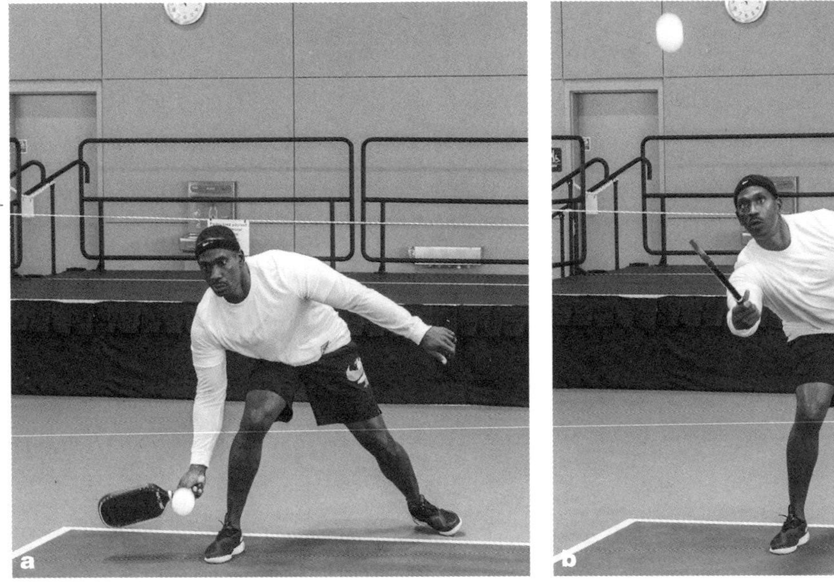

Figure 7.2 Defensive lob (*a*) lunge and contact and (*b*) follow-through.

Offensive Lob

A lob is considered offensive when it is used unexpectedly and purposefully to force the opponents into a weaker position, catching them off guard. This lob is generally used when all four players are at the NVZ and the opponents are poised for a dink or a quick attacking volley. The more deceptive you are as you execute it, the more effective it will be. Look as though you are about to hit a lower shot, but at the last instant drop your paddle on the backswing and come through with the lifting action of a good lob. Many offensive lobbers recommend aiming the lob over the backhand shoulder of one opponent, keeping the ball away from the strength of any overhead slam.

While you should hit a defensive lob quite high in the air to give yourself needed time, an offensive lob should just clear the paddle of the upward-reaching opposing player. You don't want to give your opponent time to turn and run to the ball in time to hit it, or—worse—allow them to hit a too-low lob with an attacking overhead swing that can drive the ball downward with force.

An excellent time to execute an offensive lob is off a crosscourt dink coming to your forehand side and close to that sideline. In this scenario, all four players are at the net and focused on dinking the next shot. You are to your partner's right. Your opponent (D1 in figure 7.3) hits a beautiful crosscourt dink, which lands on the sideline to your right. Even though you (L1) have to step forward and to the side to get to the ball, as you prepare to hit the ball you feel balanced and in control. Then instead of executing a crosscourt dink back across the net, you open the paddle face, sweep your paddle arm close to your body as you bring it forward, and lift the ball up and over the player directly opposite you

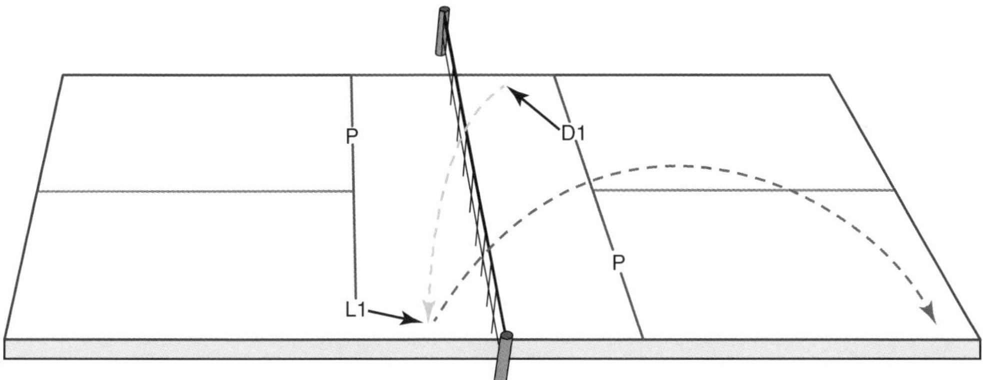

Figure 7.3 Returning the opponents' dink with a lob.

or diagonally above the space between the opponents. The ball lands near one of the back corners of the court. If your opponents are able to get to the ball, it is virtually impossible for their hit to be aggressive; most likely it will be a setup for a kill shot by your team, or at least give your team an advantage by holding the dominant position at the NVZ with your opponents forced back toward their baseline.

More to Choose and Use

DEFENDING AGAINST THE LOB

Defending against a well-hit deep lob requires excellent communication between partners. If the player over whom the ball is being lobbed can get to the ball by taking just one or two steps backward, that player should call for it—"Mine!" or "I've got it!"—turn the left side of the body to the net (for a right-handed player), take sideways steps to get into position behind the ball, and hit the ball forcefully, at a downward angle, while it's still in the air (known as an overhead smash, explained in chapter 8).

If, however, it's too deep to reach, that player (player C in figure 7.4) should let their partner know that by saying, "Yours!" or "Take it!"—anything that indicates the partner should try to get the ball. Players should *never* backpedal to get to the ball! That is an invitation for injury. In response to the instruction to take the ball, the partner (player D) then turns and runs at an angle back to the ball and returns it with a hard drive, a soft drop shot over the net, or another lob. While he is doing this, player C at the non-volley line may slide over to assume what was originally the partner's position at the non-volley line, calling, "Switch!" As soon as player D returns the lob, player D moves straight forward to the non-volley line. Players C and D are once again side by side at the non-volley line, even though they are not in their original positions.

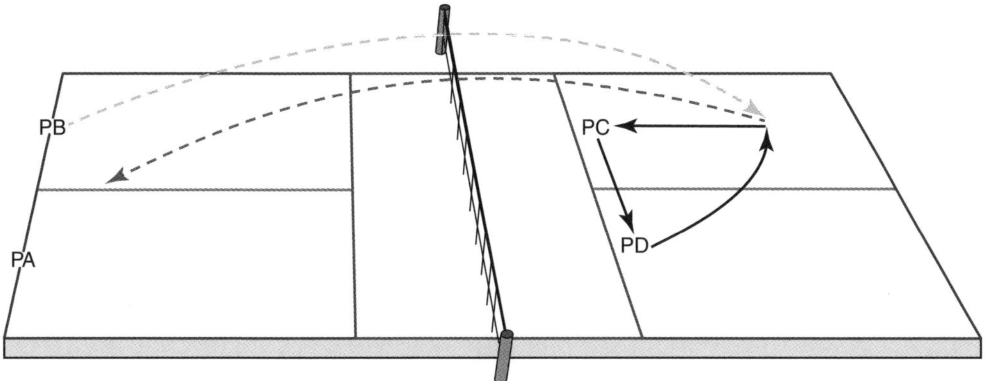

Figure 7.4 Using teamwork to defend against the lob.

They maintain these new positions until the rally is over, at which time they resume their correct (original) positions. If the lob is not deep in the back corner or the returning player is very quick on their feet, it may make sense for the partner to not call to switch sides. Some teams will play such that both players move back on a lob, then move forward together toward the net, much like how the serving team earned their way up to a strong offensive position where both players are up near the NVZ line after letting the return of serve bounce.

This defensive maneuver is much more successful if the lobbed ball goes to the deep forehand corner of the defending team's court. This allows the player who hustles back at an angle in pursuit of the ball to return the lob with a forehand shot. If, however, the lob goes to the defending team's backhand corner, the return shot may be more difficult because it must be made with a backhand stroke. As always, there are exceptions to any generality like this: some players have stronger backhands and prefer that shot. It is to all players' advantage to be aware of what shots their opponents rely on or find most comfortable. In a competitive game, it is to your advantage to place your shots away from their "comfort zone."

Take It to the Court

You might not always have a coach or veteran player available to analyze your play. Use the following information to diagnose and correct errors that you might be committing.

Lobbing the ball too shallow in the opponents' court

- *Focus on the paddle face being more behind the ball as well as under the ball at the point of ball contact.* If the paddle face is too much under the ball, the ball will travel high over the net but not very deep, providing a good setup for your opponents to execute an aggressive smash.
- *Concentrate on getting the feel of the perfectly executed lob.* The lifting action of executing a good lob requires a feel for how much force is necessary for the ball to travel high enough and deep enough to clear the opponents but still land inside the boundary lines.
- *Learn from your mistakes.* If the first lob is too shallow or too low, apply more force on the next one. If that lob is better, try to remember how it felt: the position of your body, your arm swing, the contact of the ball, and the follow-through.

Lobbing the ball too low

- *Ensure that the face of your paddle is under the ball as well as behind it.*
- *Use more force at the moment of contact with the ball.*

Missing too long

- *Think of the body action required to hit a good lob as being a lift of the ball rather than a brisk hit of the ball.*
- *Decrease the force applied to the forward swing of the paddle arm before contacting the ball.* You're hitting it too hard!

Missing to the right or to the left

- *Ensure that the face of the paddle is square to the target as the ball is contacted.*
- *Note the forward swing of your paddle arm from your right hip.* It should be in line with the target.

Give It a Go

Following are drills that players can use for the purpose of practicing the lob as well as defense of the lob. Focus on lifting the ball up and over the net and over the reach of an imaginary player on the other side.

BOUNCE AND LOB

Two players stand behind or near the baseline at opposite ends of the court, one on each side of the net, diagonally across the net from each other (figure 7.5). One player (L1) bounces the ball to themselves and lobs it over the net to the opposite deep court, where the other player (L2) catches the ball and returns it with another lob. After eight or ten lobs each, the players switch positions to hit the lobs directly across the net rather than diagonally. When lobbing, players should concentrate on lifting the ball rather than hitting it, picturing an arc over the lifted paddle of an imaginary player standing at the NVZ.

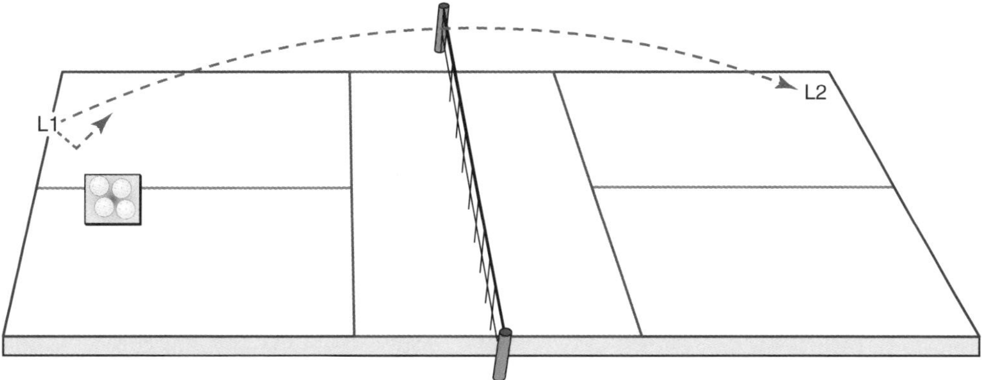

Figure 7.5 Bounce and lob drill.

THROW AND LOB

One player (L) stands near the baseline at one end of the court, on either side of the center line (figure 7.6). Directly across the net, just behind the non-volley line, stands the feeder (F). The feeder either throws or hits the ball across the net to the lobber (L), who is in a ready position, prepared to lob the ball. After sending the ball to the lobbing player, the feeder stands up straight, holding the paddle above their head. L lobs the ball over the feeder directly opposite them, aiming to clear the paddle and land deep in the court near the baseline. After 10 or so lobs, the players switch roles and repeat.

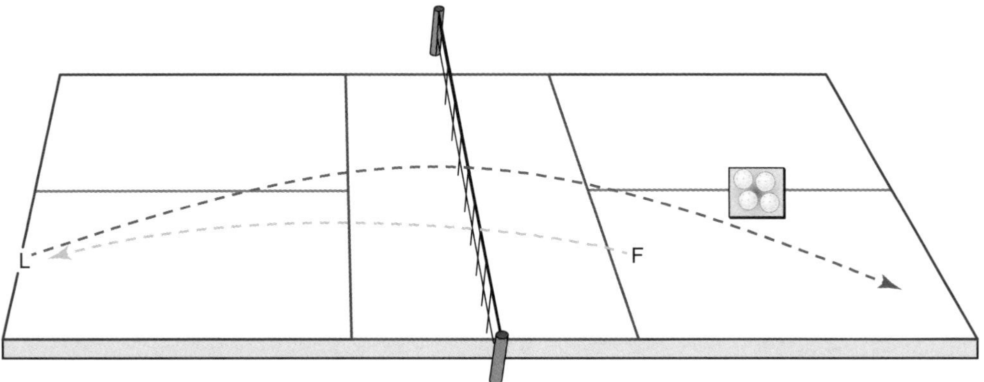

Figure 7.6 Throw and lob drill.

LOB FROM A DINK

Four players set up at the net and engage in a dink rally. As soon as the opportunity arises, D2 hits a sharp crosscourt dink to L1. Player D3 stands upright, holding the paddle overhead, as player L1 executes a lob over the top of D3's paddle (figure 7.7). After L1 has tried four or five lobs, the players rotate, so all players have an opportunity to work on lobs from this position.

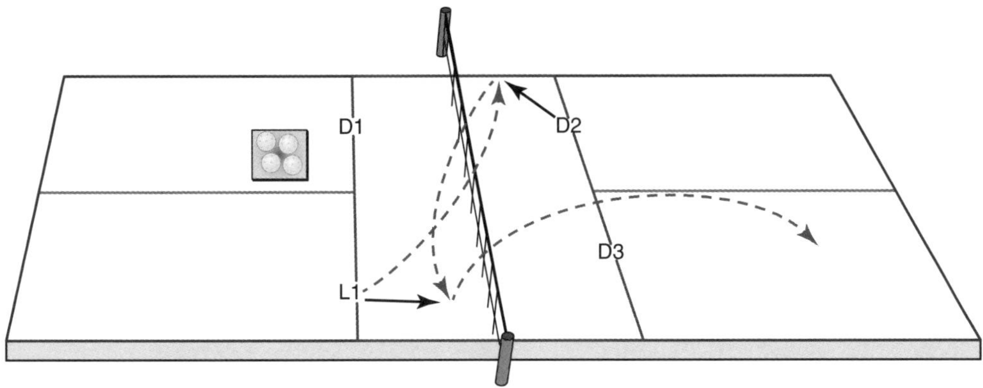

Figure 7.7 Lob from a dink drill.

SERVE, RETURN, LOB, AND RALLY

Four players get into position as if they were starting a game, S and L on the serving side and R1 and R2 on the return side. Player S serves the ball. Player R1 returns the serve slow and deep and follows it up by going to the NVZ line. The player to whom the serve return is hit (L) executes a lob, after which players S and L go to the NVZ line. The two teams play out the rally and then start the action again with another serve from S (figure 7.8). Players should rotate and also change the serve position to behind the left service court.

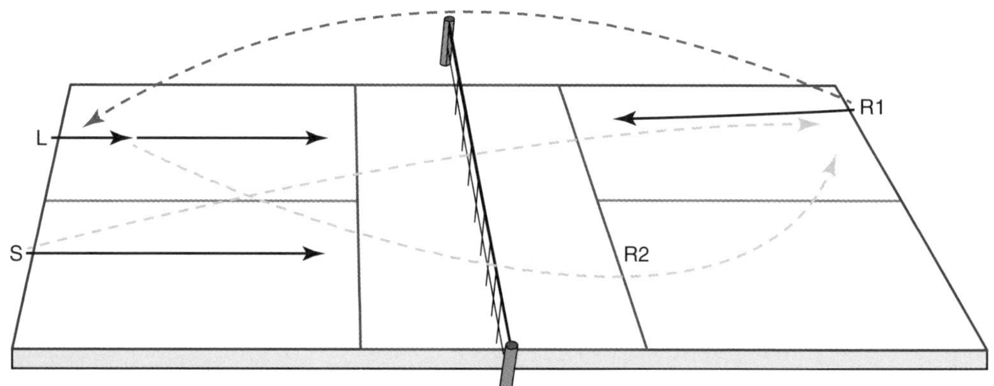

Figure 7.8 Serve, return, lob, and rally drill.

Match Point

While you can use a lob effectively in a game, you should not overuse it. It becomes evident early in some games when a team likes to lob and seems to do it endlessly. Smart opponents who see that this is happening will, instead of moving to a position close against the NVZ line, stay farther back—3 feet or so (about a meter) behind the NVZ line—so that they're in a strong position to return the lob with an offensive shot. Their objective should be to force their lobbing opponents away from their preferred shot and make them hit something else! Use the lob when you simply have no better choice or at a time when it is unexpected and difficult to return effectively.

CHAPTER

8

Overhead Smash

The overhead smash may be the most aggressive, offensive, and intimidating shot in pickleball. Usually used to return an opponent's mishit shot, such as a not-high-enough lob or any other popped-up shot, the smash is a forceful hit executed as high in the air as the player can reach and directed downward at a sharp angle into the opponents' court, ideally toward a location that is difficult to reach or return effectively. A well-executed smash can be almost impossible to defend.

You Can Do It

EXECUTING THE OVERHEAD SMASH

The overhead smash is used to return a high, lofted ball, whether it is a purposeful lob or an accidental pop-up. As soon as the ball leaves your opponent's paddle and you see that it is probably going to be a setup for an overhead smash, move to a position behind the ball. Continue to track the flight of the ball with your eyes as you move into position, being cautious to keep a balanced position to your feet and not step backwards. If it appears that the ball will be either over your head directly or slightly behind you, turn your body so that your left side (for the right-handed player) faces the net and side-step to a spot that, if you were to allow the ball to drop to the ground, it would land between you and the net and in line with your paddle arm. As you watch the ball drop down, you should be in a forward-stride position with your right foot back. Your paddle arm should be cocked behind the right shoulder with the head of the paddle back and down (figure 8.1*a*). Swing the paddle arm up and forward so that you contact the ball high in the air with arm and wrist action. The ideal position of your paddle at the time of ball contact should be behind and on the top half of the ball, driving it down at an angle. Shift your body weight from the rear foot to the forward foot as you execute the smash (8.1*b*). This adds force to the hit. After ball contact, follow through, letting your arm continue in a downward arc across your body and toward the ground (8.1*c*).

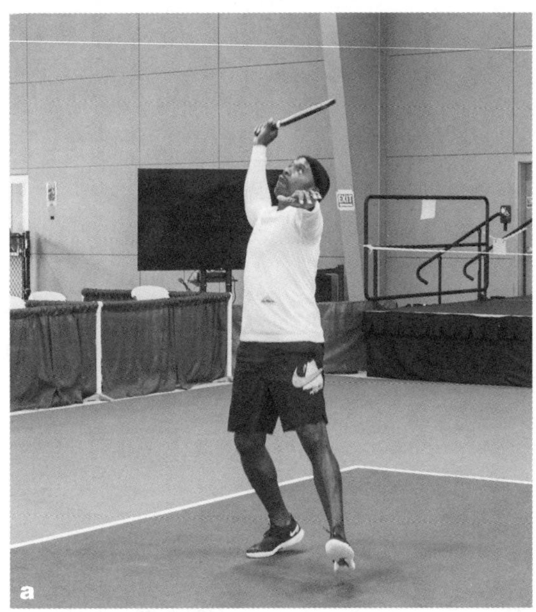

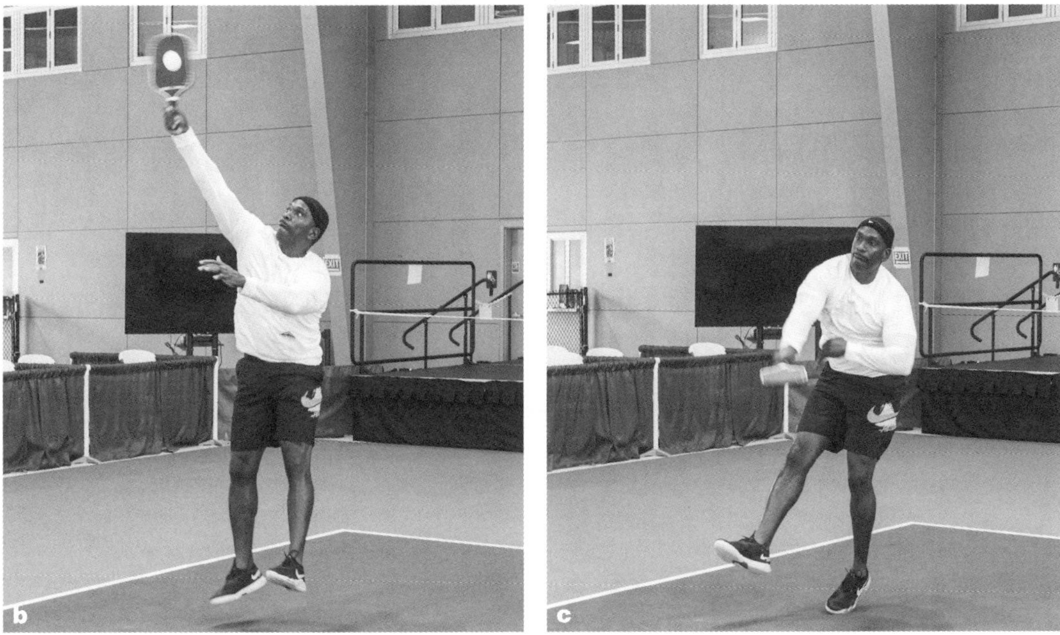

Figure 8.1 Executing a forehand overhead smash: (*a*) preparation, (*b*) contact, and (*c*) follow-through.

The closer you are to the non-volley line, the sharper the downward angle that you can put on your hit by placing the paddle more on top of the ball (figure 8.2). If you're deeper in the court, you need to keep your paddle more behind the ball than on top of it for your hit to clear the net.

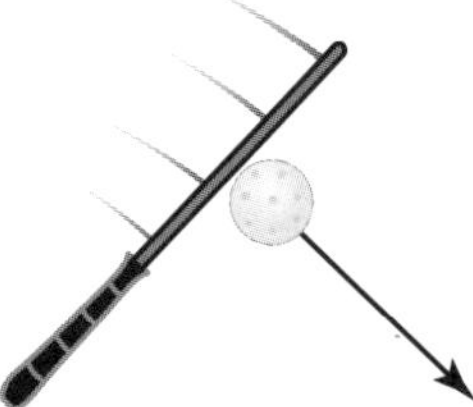

Figure 8.2 Paddle position for executing the overhead smash.

As you learn and practice the overhead smash, remember the rules pertaining to the non-volley zone (NVZ). Any shot after the serve—whether it is a dink, smash, drop, drive, or lob—hit before the ball bounces is a volley. No part of your body, your equipment, or your clothing can contact the NVZ, including the lines denoting the boundaries of the zone, during any part of the volley and including the follow-through. Even if the ball is dead in the opponent's court, this rule applies to any momentum from executing the volley. Refer to the *International Federation of Pickleball Official Tournament Rulebook* (usapickleball.org) for details; it is updated annually.

Because there can be a lot of adrenaline flowing when you see a perfect setup for a smash, it's easy to forget where you are on the court! It would not be a happy moment if, after executing the perfect smash, you were called for a line violation because your momentum carried you into the NVZ. Know where you are on the court at all times. Also, because of the exhilaration that comes with seeing that perfect setup, it is important to communicate early and clearly with your partner as to who will hit the smash. Otherwise the two of you may both swing hard, possibly smashing a finger, clashing paddles, or hitting a fault instead of an easy "winner."

More to Choose and Use

BACKHAND SMASH

Most overhead smashes are executed on the forehand side of the body. You could execute a backhand smash, but it would have less force coming from that side (figure 8.3). Hitting the ball overhead with any downward force using your backhand requires a backward flexing of the wrist, which is not easy for many people without practice. Whenever possible, you should slide to the side as the ball comes toward you so that you can use your forehand when executing a smash. Fortunately, a high, lofted shot ideal for a smash allows extra time for this adjustment in positioning as well as clear partner communication like "Mine!" or "Take it!"

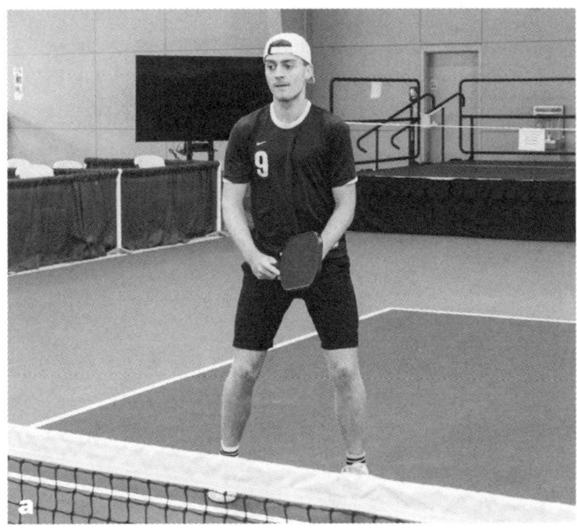

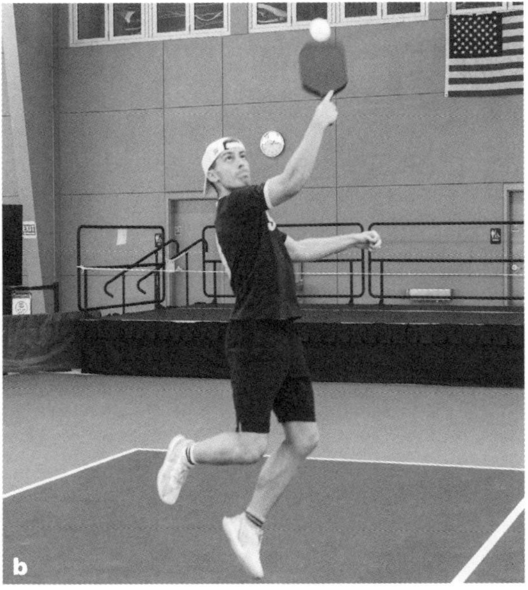

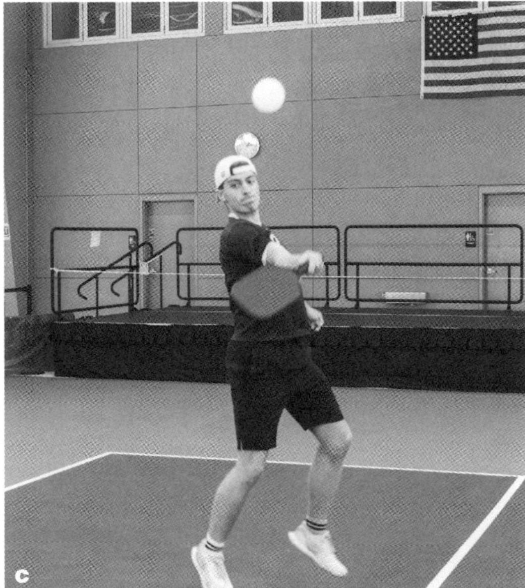

Figure 8.3 Executing a backhand overhead smash: (*a*) preparation, (*b*) contact, and (*c*) follow-through.

DEFENDING AGAINST THE SMASH

If your reaction time is quick enough and you are in a good ready position, you might be able to get your paddle on a ball that is smashed for a return volley. Simply blocking, with no swing, the force of the ball as it contacts your paddle can cause the ball to rebound back over the net. It is much easier, though, to contact the smash after it has bounced, slowing the ball down and giving you more reaction time.

In either situation it is important that is that you and your partner, upon seeing that one of you has just hit a ball that is a perfect setup for a smashed ball coming back at you, move back in your court if at all possible. If you're still at the NVZ line and the ball is hit hard right at you, there is less chance that you can react fast enough to get your paddle on it and send it back across the net. However, if you're deeper in your court, you have more time to react and at least have a chance at getting your paddle on the ball for a controlled return. It is crucial that you and your partner communicate with each other and react to each other's movements and that you do it quickly. Sometimes you may only have time to take a single step back and attempt a block; at other times, a high, lofted shot will allow you time to move back near the baseline, poised to move to each side and take the smash off the bounce. If you are at the baseline and the smash will not bounce before it reaches you, just let it go: a bounce behind the baseline is a fault, an "out" ball, giving you an easy way to win that rally. One of the biggest differences between the most successful players and others is their ability to quickly decide to let "out" balls go and resist the urge to hit them.

Take It to the Court

The ability to correct your own errors is crucial to your consistent success on a pickleball court. Don't be content committing the same error over and over. The following information will help you to pinpoint the cause of your error and then help you correct it.

Hitting the ball into the net

- *Be patient!* Watch the ball strike the paddle and keep your head up while hitting. Rushing the shot, looking down too early, and being too anxious can result in an erratic hit.
- *Be sure that the face of the paddle is behind and on top of the ball on contact.* Placing the paddle's impact point too much on top of the ball can cause it to go down and into the net.

Missing too long to the right or to the left

- *Aim your smash down the middle of the court or to the opponents' feet.* Don't try for a perfect smash right on the sideline.
- *Think of your hit being half speed instead of trying to kill the ball.* A well-placed, controlled smash can be just as effective as a hard-hit one.

Limited force on the ball

- *Focus on slowing down your total action.* Rushing the shot will sometimes cause the contact to be made close to the edge of the paddle rather than in the sweet spot.
- *Practice the smash with someone throwing the ball to you until your timing is perfect.* Think more about placement and success than the speed of the hit.
- *Balance and position yourself behind the ball properly before striking the overhead ball.*

Give It a Go

Following are some drills that you can use for practicing the smash. Strive for patience as the lofted ball drops into position for your smash.

THROW AND SMASH

On the left side of the net, one player (OS) stands in the middle of the service box, ready to execute an overhead smash. Across the net, a feeder (F) is at the NVZ court with a supply of balls. The feeder throws a high, lofted ball to OS, who smashes it back. The throw should be underhand. If it's easier for the feeders to hit rather than throw the ball to initiate play, that's fine. This drill can also be done with two OS, each in one of the two service boxes on the left side of the net, hitting overheads from either one or two feeders (figure 8.4).

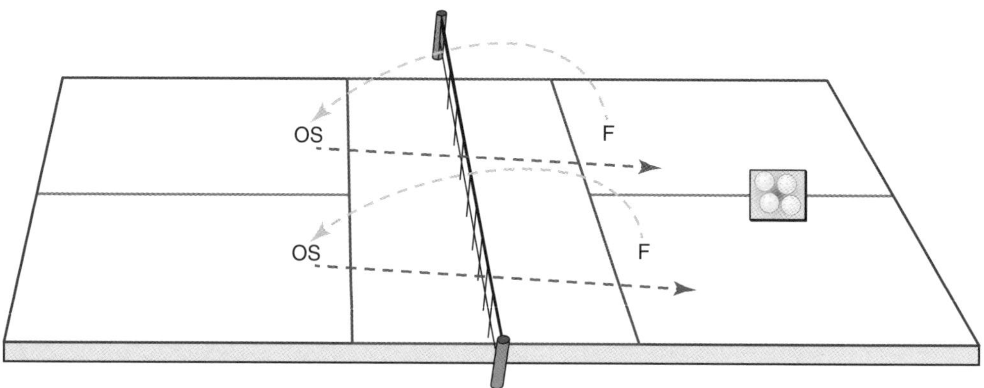

Figure 8. 4 Throw and smash drill.

LOB AND SMASH

One player (OS) sets up at the non-volley line on the right side of the net. OS hits a groundstroke across the net to L. L lobs the ball over OS, trying to keep it within reach of OS's overhead swing. OS smashes it back to L, who tries to keep the rally going by lobbing it again. If it is not possible for L to execute another lob, play begins again, with OS hitting the groundstroke to L. If the drill is done with two OS players on left and right sides of the NVZ line (figure 8.5), they should alternate starting the play so that no one gets hit by a smashed ball. After a few rallies, players can rotate positions on the court so that all players get a turn to lob and to smash.

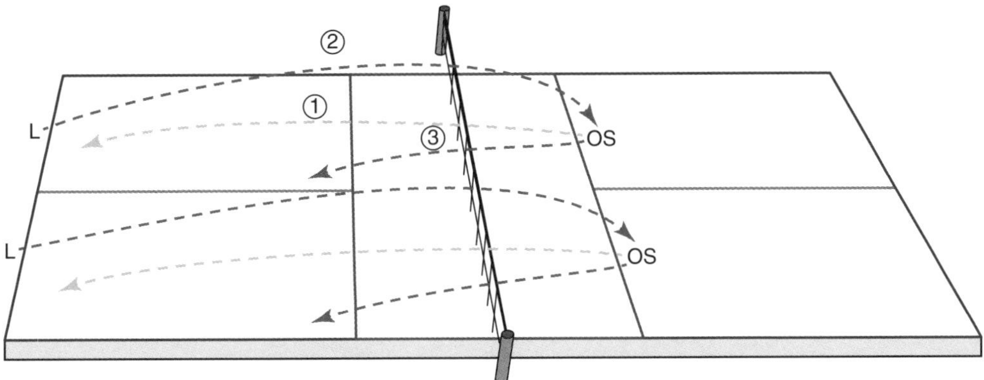

Figure 8.5 Lob and smash drill.

HOT POTATO

On the left side of the net, two players (F1 and F2) stand in the middle of each half court with three balls in their hands. On the right side of the net, two players (P1 and P2) wait at the NVZ line in their half of the court. Each feeder tosses one ball just over the net, which the opposing player dinks back. Each feeder then tosses a setup for a low volley, which the player across the net volleys back. Each feeder then tosses a lob, which the opposing player smashes (figure 8.6). After the first three balls are thrown and returned, the sequence of tosses should change so that the players can't anticipate which type of shot will be required but must react to the type of ball that is thrown. After a few series of tosses, players rotate positions on the court so that all players have the opportunity to hit the hot potato. This drill can be done with one feeder and one receiving player or with two receivers alternating.

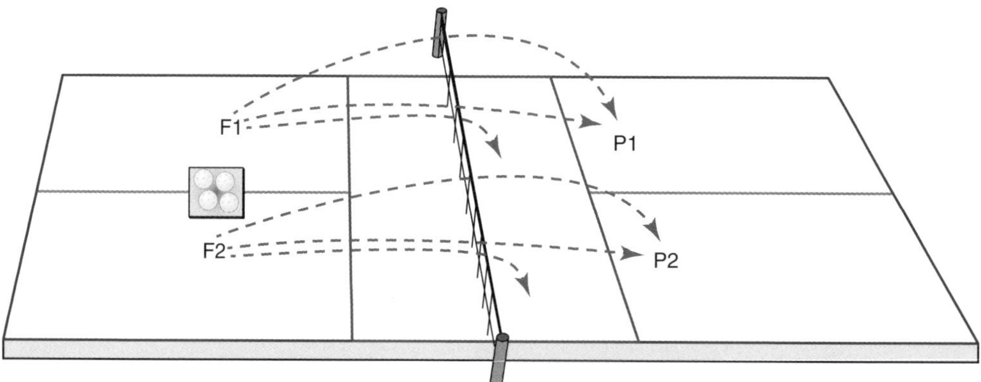

Figure 8.6 Hot potato drill.

Match Point

The overhead smash, or any other related shot that allows you to drive a high ball downward with force, is a reliable rally winner in a pickleball game. Whenever the opportunity presents itself during a rally, smash the ball back, downward and with force. The soft net game of successive dinks is a vital part of the game, but an important goal should always be to take advantage of the dink or another shot that your opponent hits too high by smashing it back. As much as possible, you want to force your opponent to hit their shots upward over the net (as after a shot hit low, near their feet) while you are looking for every opportunity to hit your shots downward. Always maintain your cool at the net. Be patient and controlled and you will win games!

CHAPTER

9

Drop Shot

A drop shot is usually hit off a bounce from deep in the court, softly arcing the ball into the non-volley zone (NVZ) so that the opponents have little opportunity for a quick offensive shot. It may be considered a "dink in a different direction" since the ball follows a similar arcing flight, but it is hit from farther back in the court rather than close to the NVZ line.

While the body position of the player hitting the drop shot resembles that of a player hitting a groundstroke, the forward swing of the paddle arm is slower, with more lift. The object of hitting a drop shot is to give the team deep in their court—usually the serving team—the opportunity to safely follow the shot up to the NVZ line. A drop shot should have a somewhat lofted trajectory, with the high point of the arch being over the hitting player's NVZ. When hit correctly, the ball will drop over the net and land softly in or very near the opponent's NVZ.

A typical rally in a well-played pickleball game is likely to include the initial serve that lands deep in the court diagonally across from the server; the second shot, a return of the serve that is high and deep, giving the serve receiver time to get to the NVZ line to join their partner; and the third, a drop shot hit by a player on the serving team. That drop shot is then followed up with both partners moving with quick but controlled steps to the NVZ line. Not every good rally will follow this exact pattern, but many will. A common variation is when the return of serve is hit short, and the serving team chooses to take advantage of this by moving forward and driving the third shot hard and low with topspin, either between the opponents or directly at them, giving them little time to react.

You Can Do It

EXECUTING THE DROP SHOT

Learning to execute a consistently good drop shot is not easy, but the time and effort devoted to perfecting it is well worth it at game time. It provides a team that has been forced deep in their court with a means to get to the net, safe from most offensive attack shots. In a game, it is commonly the serving team that utilizes the first drop shot of a rally, to the extent that many players call it a 'third-shot drop."

A drop shot can also be effective if your opponents are both deep in their court or if one player is up and the other is back. In either case, placing the ball just over the net in an open space can be a rally winner (figure 9.1).

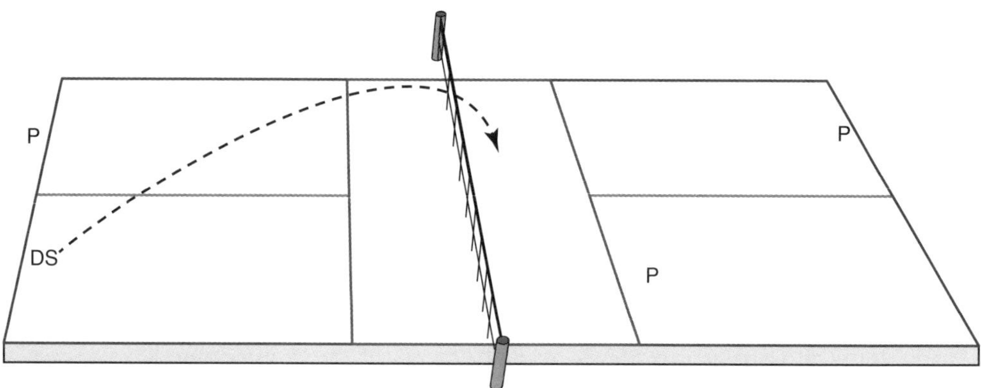

Figure 9.1 Hitting the drop shot into open space.

The most widely used return of a good drop shot is a dink. Because the dink is a softly hit shot that takes some time to cross the net and land in your opponents' court, it gives you and your partner time to move toward the NVZ line.

As the ball is coming toward you, move to it as if you were going to return it with a groundstroke. Take short, comfortable steps to a position behind and to the left (for the right-hander) of the bouncing ball, keeping the ball between you and the net and to the right and in front of your right knee (figure 9.2*a*). Your weight should be balanced on both feet and your body facing the right net post. As you move the paddle back in preparation for the forward swing, open the face of the paddle slightly. From the moment you start the forward swing of the paddle arm, you should focus on a soft, controlled contact of the ball (9.2*b*). The face of the paddle should be behind and slightly below the ball at the point of contact, and your weight should shift from the rear foot to the forward foot. After contact, follow through toward the target (9.2*c*). The flight of the ball as it travels forward should gently loft.

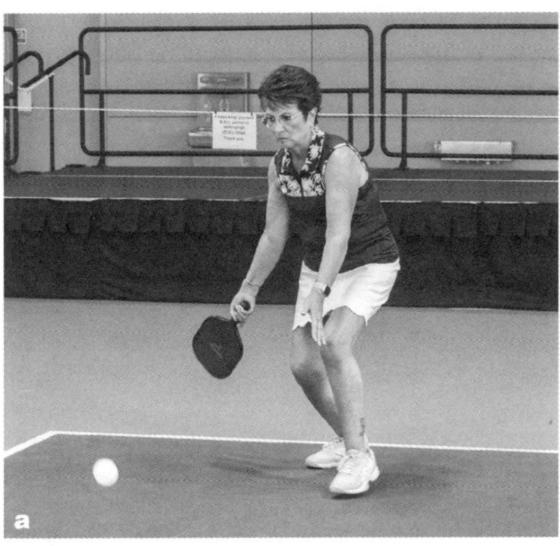

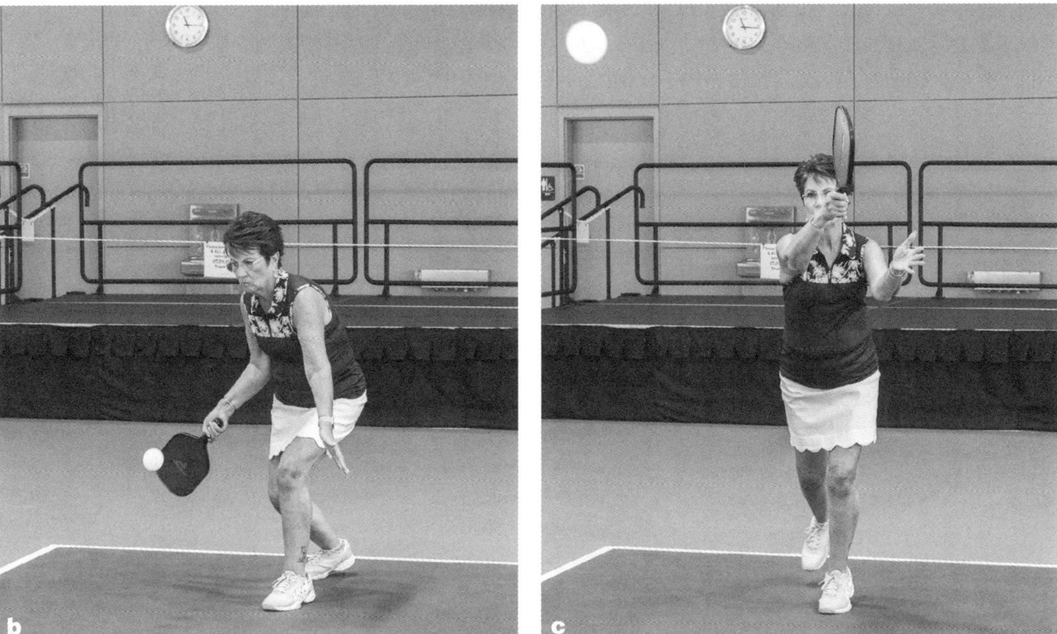

Figure 9.2 Executing the drop shot: (*a*) preparation, (*b*) contact, and (*c*) follow-through.

Your objective is to hit the ball so that the highest point of its arc is over your side of the net, fairly close to the NVZ. The ball should then drop down into the opponents' NVZ, softly enough that it won't bounce up high enough to be effectively attacked (figure 9.3). Most important when executing a drop shot is that it be soft and controlled!

Does much of this description sound familiar? It should, from the chapter on dinks. After all, a drop shot truly is often a "dink in another direction."

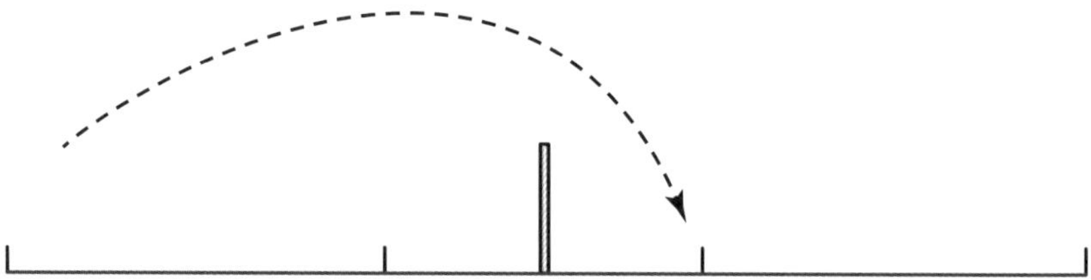

Figure 9.3 Flight path of drop shot.

If you have trouble executing a drop shot from the baseline, try practicing from midcourt. As you're able, move back gradually until you're at the baseline. Give yourself room: the ball does not need to just barely miss the top of the net and it doesn't need to land as close to the net as possible. Many players have trouble with a soft shot dropping right toward their feet, so that can make a good target for aiming your shot. If you aim to just barely miss the net top, you're thinking about the net, and that's a good way to hit your shot into the net. Instead, pick a target that you do want to hit, like an opponent's backhand foot or a spot slightly inside the NVZ line in front of their feet. These are locations where the opponent will need to make a quick choice to either reach out awkwardly to hit the drop low in front of them (which would be a volley, forcing them to avoid the NVZ), or wait for it to bounce at their feet, possibly forcing them to step back away from the NVZ line.

Both of their options are defensive, upward shots. Putting your opponents where they must make a rapid decision like this only increases their chance of making a mistake, faulting into the net, or popping up their return for an easy put-away smash for your team.

More to Choose and Use

DEFENDING AGAINST THE DROP SHOT

The players on the serve-receive team can often tell by looking at the player who is about to contact the ball on the serving team what kind of shot that player will hit. Body position, the position of the paddle, and the aggressiveness of backswing and body movement may indicate whether the intended shot is a drop shot, a groundstroke, or a lob. If the backswing and movement are slow and gentle, the player is likely preparing to hit a drop shot. If they move their paddle toward the ground, the intended shot is probably a lob, and if they rear back with an aggressive backswing and use a wider stance of the feet, expect a hard-driving groundstroke. Be prepared for the intended shot coming to you by paying attention to the total action of the opposing player preparing to hit the ball.

Take It to the Court

The drop shot, which can be difficult to execute, is also important for you to master. Being able to correct your own errors will speed up that process. Here are some common errors and tips for correcting them.

The ball goes into the net

- *Concentrate on not stopping the forward motion of the paddle arm. Remember to open the face of the paddle before and during contact with the ball.*
- *Make it your objective to have enough net clearance and for the ball to land softly, close to your opponent's feet or to their backhand near the NVZ line.* By giving them a shot that lands softly and doesn't bounce high, your opponents can't do much with it except dink it back.

The ball goes too deep and too high, giving your opponent a good setup for an offensive downward shot

- *Soften your hit by slowing down your swing or shortening the backswing, being sure your arm is pivoting at the shoulder, neither wrist nor elbow moving much, if at all.*
- *Execute a drop shot only if you are in a balanced, controlled position.* Don't try for one if you're on the defensive, struggling to get to the ball, or lunging for the ball.

You miss either to the right or to the left

- *Aim for the center of the court at first rather than trying to make the shot too precisely near the sidelines.* The net is lower in the middle of the court than at the sidelines—34 inches (86 cm) in the middle and 36 inches (91 cm) at the sidelines—so it's also an easier shot to make.
- *Be in complete control and balanced before you attempt to execute a drop shot.* If you're not, your shot can be erratic. Use an elongated motion with the paddle face going towards the intended target to ensure better directional control.

Give It a Go

The following drills are for two players or more for the practice of the drop shot. These drills progress from fairly simple to more complicated and difficult. Don't be intimidated by them. Be persistent and patient and you will discover positive carryover from the drills to your next game. That will make your day!

SELF-BOUNCE AND DROP SHOT

A player (DS) stands behind the baseline with a ball hopper or supply of balls close at hand. They bounce a ball and then hit a drop shot arcing over the net, aiming to land it near the opposite NVZ line. After completing several drop shots, the player then alternates between hitting a groundstroke (driven harder, aiming close to the far baseline) and hitting a drop shot off the bounce (figure 9.4). The player should concentrate on feeling the difference between hitting a hard groundstroke and hitting a softly arcing drop shot. Two players can practice this at the same time, both positioned behind the same baseline. For greater challenge as skills progress, this same drill can be done by tossing the ball up somewhat randomly, then quickly moving to a position behind where the ball will bounce and executing the drop shot from there.

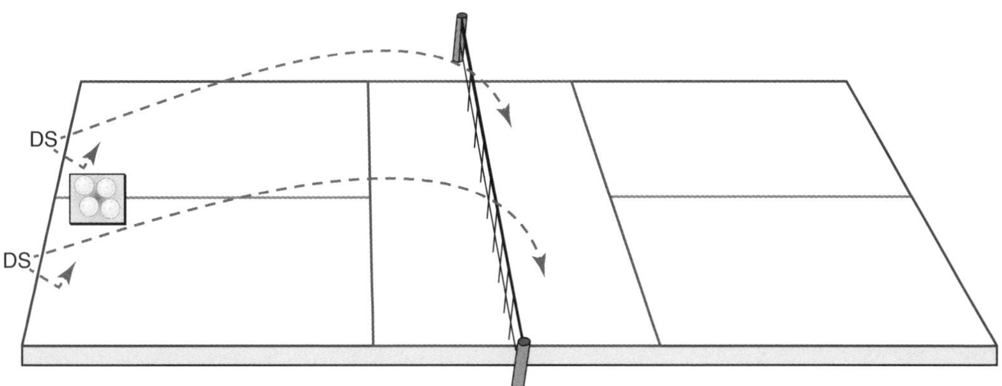

Figure 9.4 Self-bounce and drop shot drill.

THROW AND DROP SHOT

One or two feeders (F) stand in either half of the court on the left side of the net with a supply of balls close at hand. One or two players (DS) stand at the baseline in either half of the court on the right side of the net. The feeders throw balls to the players across the net; players hit the ball after the bounce with a drop shot (figure 9.5). For added challenge, place a target in the middle of the court that is as high as the net (a tall box works well) and keep track of the number of drop shots that hit or enter the target. Players rotate so that feeders, too, have the opportunity to hit drop shots.

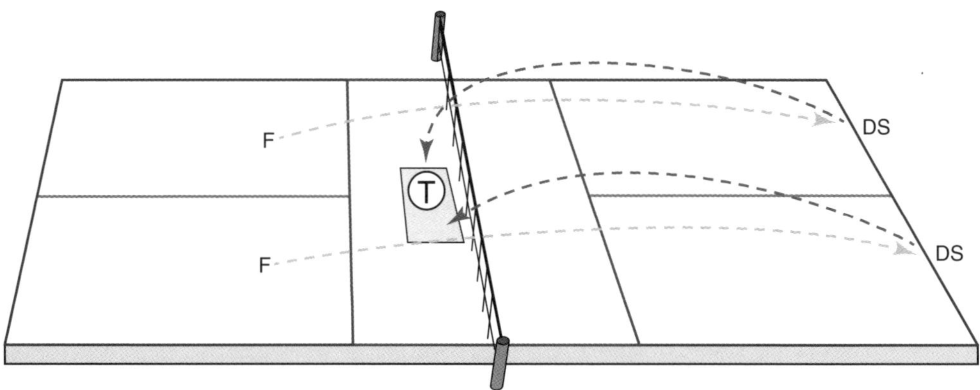

Figure 9.5 Throw and drop shot drill.

HARD AND SOFT

On the left side of the net, one or two feeders (F) stand in each half of the court with a supply of balls at hand. Across the net from each feeder, a player (DS) stands at the baseline. The feeders throw balls to the players across the net; players alternate between hitting a hard groundstroke and hitting a soft drop shot. Hitters should get a feel for the difference between hitting a hard groundstroke and hitting a soft, arcing drop shot (figure 9.6). Players rotate positions so that all have the opportunity to practice the shots.

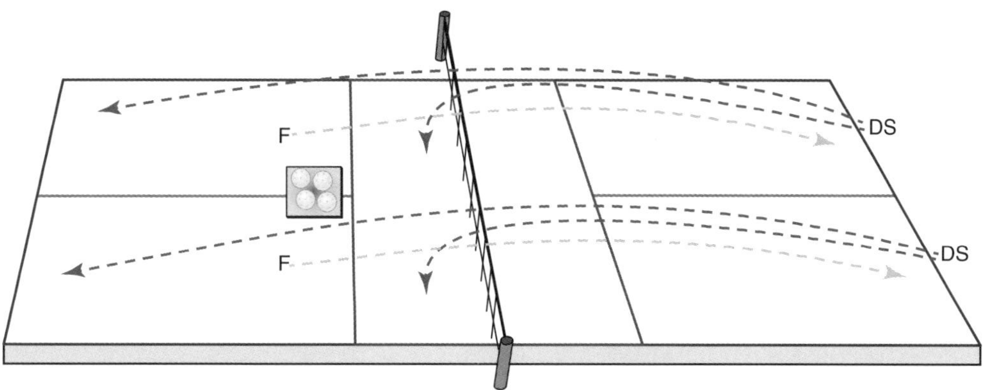

Figure 9.6 Hard and soft drill.

CHECK IT

The saying "practice makes perfect" is not necessarily true. During practice, if you emphasize correct execution while simulating a game, then there should be carryover into the actual game. But how do you know that? You can use the following checklist (figure 9.7) to evaluate execution of skills in a game. A coach or player watches one player in the game and records 1 point for every good shot and 0 for every error. At the end of the game, you can calculate totals as well as percentages. Use this chart periodically for assessing players' progress in decreasing or eliminating errors. The person completing the checklist can evaluate all the skills on the list or only the skills the player is currently working on.

Figure 9.7 Execution Checklist

Evaluator: Record 1 point for every good shot and 0 for every unforced error in each area evaluated, and record the total number of shots taken. To calculate the percentage of good shots, divide the number of good shots by the total number of shots taken, and convert the decimal result to a percentage by multiplying it by 100.

Player name:

Evaluator:

Date of evaluation:

Skill being evaluated	**Good shots**	**Errors**	**Shots taken**	**Percentage**
Serve				
Forehand groundstroke				
Backhand groundstroke				
Volley				
Dink				
Lob				
Overhead smash				
Drop shot				
Total				

Match Point

The ability to execute and use a good drop shot to gain a strong position with your partner at the NVZ is a key skill that separates the good players from the mediocre players. Too often, beginning players are content to stand deep in their court and bang the ball back and forth. Be persistent in learning the soft game—the drop shot and dink—along with getting a feel for when to effectively leave those soft shots and attack, and you'll discover the joy of playing a game that requires some real finesse. As much fun as it is to slam an overhead smash past your opponents, it's even more fun to see their faces when a well-placed slow shot leaves them off balance and defenseless. Challenge yourself to become a true competitor on the pickleball court who can successfully adjust their tactics depending on their opponents' strengths, using a full range of shots, angles, and speeds.

CHAPTER

10

Shot Selection and the Mental Game

As in any other racket or paddle sport that includes a net, a game of pickleball involves players selecting and adjusting their shot based on the speed, timing, and direction of the hit coming to them from the other side of the net as well as their opponents' positions on the court. While very few rallies in a pickleball game are exactly the same, there is an initial pattern of shots that produces an exciting and varied offensive exchange between the teams. If you wish to become a competitive player, you must become familiar with this sequence. Of course, this information is of little value unless the players on the court are able to control the direction and speed of the ball coming off the paddle. First things first! Practice each shot in the total game over and over until you are confident that, when called on to use the shot in a game, you can execute it with good control.

You Can Do It

IDEAL SHOT SEQUENCE

The following sequence of shots is ideal because it provides a means for all four players—two from the serving team and two from the receiving team—to get to the NVZ. Most rallies are won and points are scored from this position near the net—not from the baseline or from midcourt, the area between the baseline and the NVZ line (often called "no-man's-land" or the "transition zone" as a reminder that it's not a place you want to stay).

If focusing on the total sequence is too much for you to handle at first, just work on one phase. For example, work first on serving, then on returning the serve deep and slow, and finally on making the third shot, which is most often a drop shot. The third shot will determine whether the serving team can get to the net safely and consequently has a fair chance at winning the rally. If you haven't gained confidence in your drop shot, you might hit a low, hard groundstroke (the "drive") down the middle or down the sideline as a passing shot, or hit a lob. You have to put the serve-receiving team on the defensive (where they're hitting a low drop shot upward or reacting to an unexpected drive or lob) to enable you and your partner to get safely near the NVZ. If you try this too soon, without putting them on defense, they can go on the offense and attack with a strong volley at your feet, between you and your partner, or down one of the sidelines.

FIRST SHOT: SERVING TEAM

The first shot of any rally is the *serve*. Regardless of the method of serving that you decide to use, your objective is to serve the ball into the proper court over the net and inbounds, ideally deep. Once you're able to do that consistently, then you can focus on being more aggressive with your serve by aiming for the deep backhand corner, dropping it short to the outside corner, or putting spin on the ball. A deep serve will keep the player receiving the serve back in their court and farther from the net. After the serve, you and your partner should stay back, close to the baseline, in a good position to return the ball after the bounce (figure 10.1).

Try hitting serves with both forehand and backhand swings and both drop ("bounce") and traditional serves.

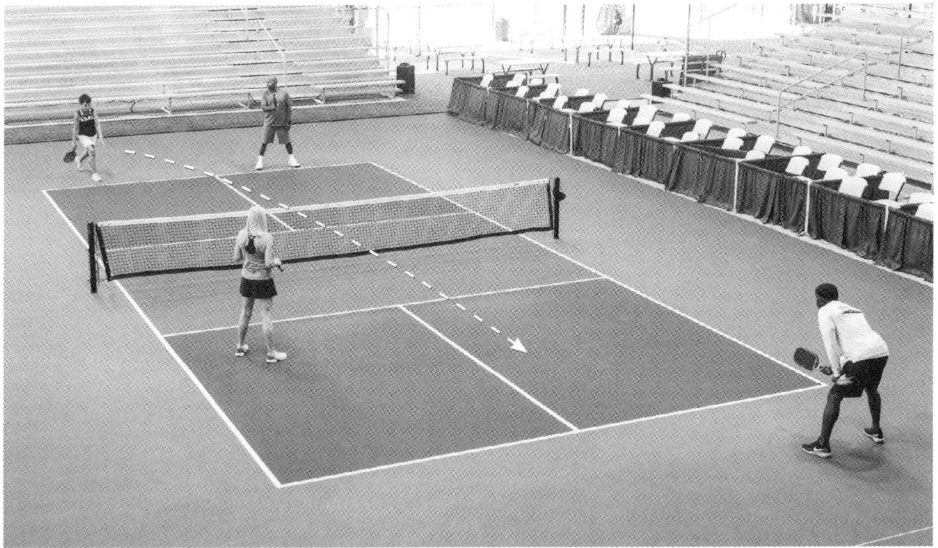

Figure 10.1 First shot: serve.

SECOND SHOT: RECEIVING TEAM

The second shot of any rally is the *return of the serve*. The ideal return of a serve for the beginning player is a hit that is slow and deep into the serving team's court (figure 10.2). Hitting it slow gives you time to follow up your shot by quickly moving forward to the NVZ line so that you're side by side with your partner in a strong offensive position (figure 10.3). To hit a slow shot that also goes deep in the opposing court, you loft the ball, arcing it over the net rather than driving it low and hard. Return the serve deep to keep the serving team back in their court.

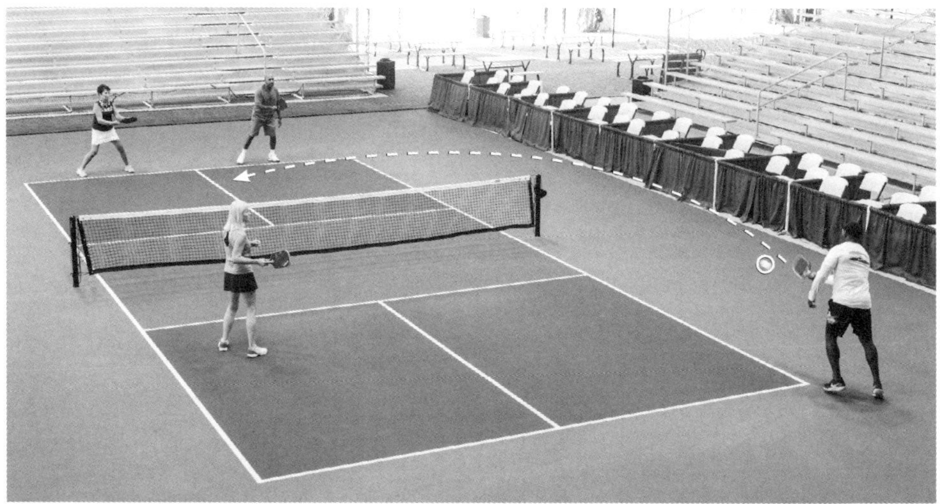

Figure 10.2 Second shot: receiving team returning the serve.

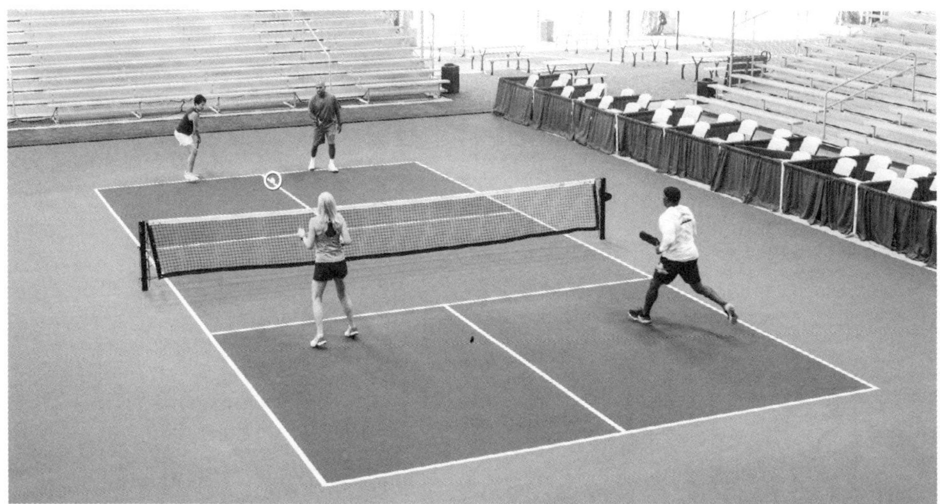

Figure 10.3 Serving team preparing to hit the third shot.

THIRD SHOT: SERVING TEAM

The third shot of any rally—the second shot hit by the serving team—determines which doubles team will gain the advantage in that particular rally. At this point, the receiving team is or should be in the NVZ—an offensive position—and the serving team is still deep in their court—a defensive position. This ensures the return bounces before they hit it, satisfying the two-bounce rule. Here are your options:

- A drop shot that arcs, landing softly over the net, with you and your partner following it up to the NVZ line, knowing the opponents will need to hit their next shot at an upward angle, most likely a dink (figure 10.4*a*).
- A hard groundstroke (drive) down the middle or near one of the outside lines, which you hope causes enough hesitation for your opponents that you and your partner can get to the net without facing an effective attacking shot. If they pop it up, you may get an easy put-away smash, or you may need to use another drop or two from inside the "transition zone" as you earn your way up to the NVZ if they are able to block the hard drive back (10.4*b*).
- A lob that forces the serve-receiving team to move back, away from the net, and allows your team to get to the NVZ line (10.4*c*) It is difficult to hit consistent, effective lobs from deep in the court, so use this third option sparingly, if at all. As discussed in chapter 7, lobs are most powerful when used unexpectedly from near the NVZ.

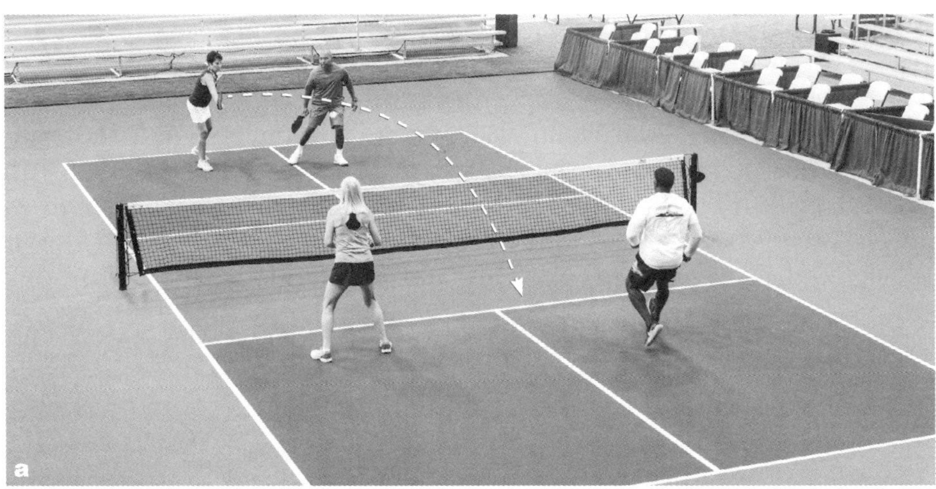

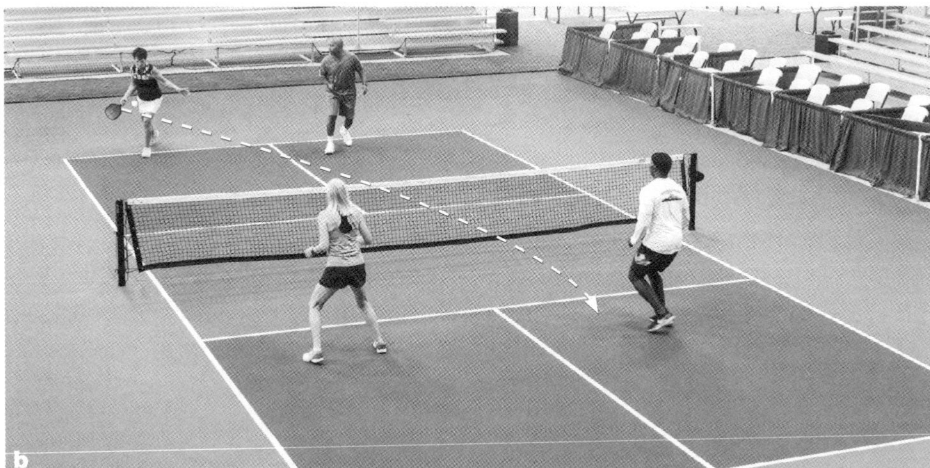

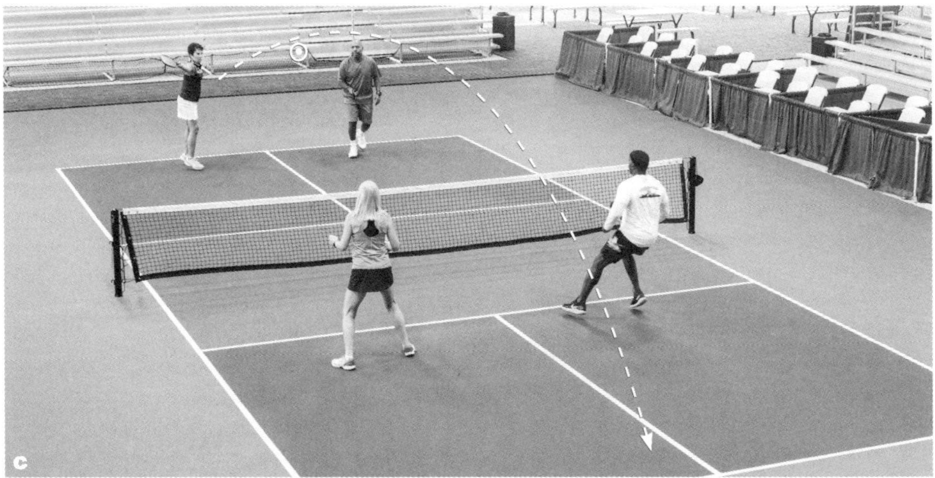

Figure 10.4 Options for third shot: (*a*) drop shot just over the net, (*b*) hard groundstroke down the middle, or (*c*) lob that forces receiving team deep.

The serving team's main objective (figure 10.5) when hitting the third shot is for it to limit the opponents' offensive choices enough to allow their own team to get to the NVZ and assume a strong, balanced ready position in time to return the next shot hit to them.

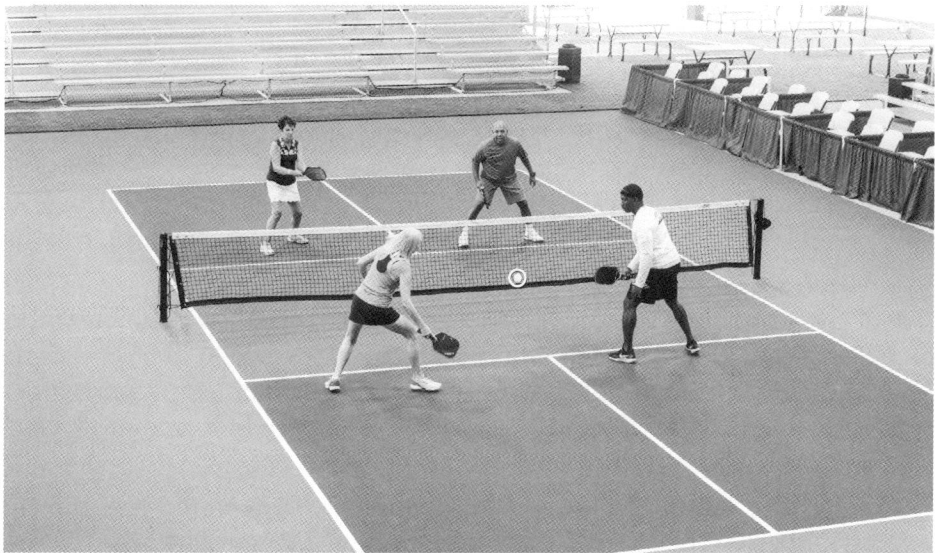

Figure 10.5 The desired result of the third shot is to allow the serving team to get to the NVZ, removing their opponents' advantage gained by reaching this spot first.

FOURTH SHOT: RECEIVING TEAM

This shot is completely dependent on what type of shot the serving team makes on the third shot.

- If the third shot is a good drop shot, the fourth shot would most likely be a dink. All four players are now at the net, looking to find or create an opening for an effective offensive attacking shot while not giving that sort of opening to the opposition. This can be the beginning of the classic "dinking duel," which can go on for many soft, slow, strategic shots, most often between two players who are diagonal from one another. Patience is a virtue here: you should try to pounce on any opportunity without rushing into an unforced error.
- If the third shot is a drive down the middle, the fourth shot would likely be a block or swinging volley. A block is likely to be returned by a short fifth-shot drop shot from the transition zone, perhaps a short hop "half-volley" of a ball hit toward the feet, leading to the same situation as above.
- If the third shot is a deep lob, the fourth shot would most likely be either a groundstroke after retreating to near the baseline or another lob off the bounce. If the serving team's third-shot lob is too short, it may well be smashed downward on the fourth shot for a rally winner.

Figure 10.6 shows the progression of the first four shots of a rally.

Figure 10.6 First Four Shots of a Rally

Shot number	Team	Type of shot		
1	Serving	Deep serve		
2	Receiving	Slow, deep return		
3	Serving	Drop	Groundstroke	Lob
4	Receiving	Dink	Volley	Groundstroke or lob

Even though the ideal is for all four players to wage this battle near the net, some players resist moving up to the NVZ (or retreat from there) for whatever reason—lack of mobility, discomfort with being too close to the action, lack of controlled aggression, or just being content to stay back and hit the ball back and forth. If you are happy playing that kind of game and you're able to find other players who are also happy to do so, then so be it. But if you truly want to become a better pickleball player and learn to play a competitive game, you have to be willing to devote the time and energy to learning and then applying some form of this three-shot sequence. A player who understands and can effectively use this sequence is also in the best position to see when an exception can be made, utilizing an unexpected shot to catch opponents by surprise.

More to Choose and Use

CAPITALIZE ON AN OPPONENT IN A VULNERABLE POSITION

If the ideal doesn't occur on the court and one or both of the players on the serving team stay back by their baseline, either by choice or because they haven't been able to return the ball with enough control to enable them to get to the net, how can the receiving team take advantage of the situation?

Dave Zapatka, an experienced tennis player and a master strategist in pickleball, answers that question this way:

> *The obvious strategy is to pin the player who remains back at the baseline back there by simply hitting deep balls in his part of the court until you're able to angle a shot between the players or to the sideline (figure 10.7). If both of them are back, you should hit deep balls anywhere in the court, pinning them both back at their baseline. This opens up the court for you to hit sharp, angled winners, overheads, and other winning shots where the ball is simply put away or dropped short out of their reach.*

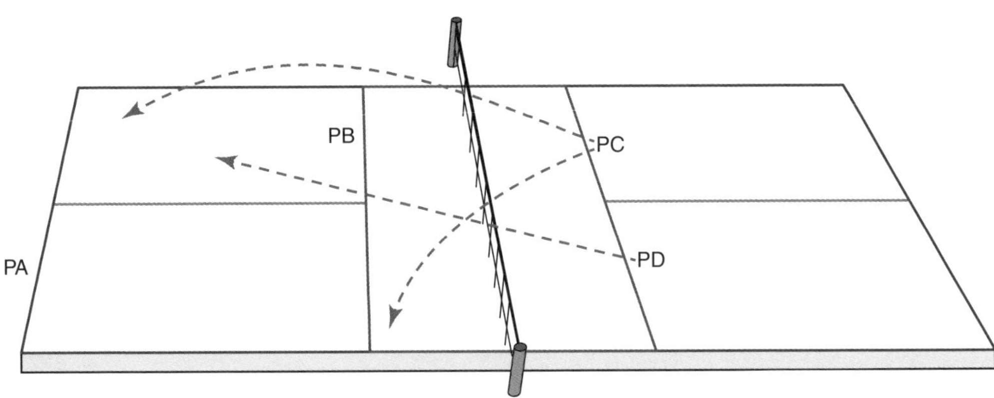

Figure 10.7 Areas of vulnerability when one opposing player is at the net and one is at the baseline.

Dave points out the pitfalls of being unable to move up to the net:

Players remaining at the baseline or in no-man's-land are vulnerable to having balls hit at their feet (figure 10.8). This, of course, puts them at a disadvantage because they always have to hit the ball upward, from below the height of the net, allowing opportunities for the opponents to hit an aggressive shot downward and once again take control of the point.

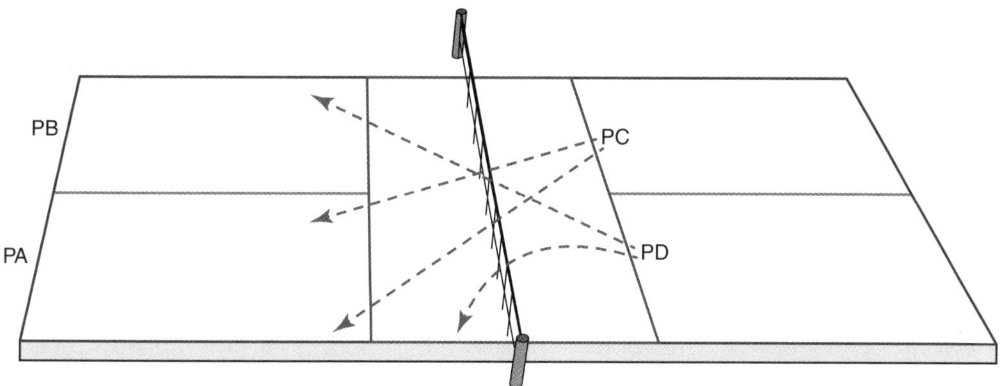

Figure 10.8 Areas of vulnerability when both opposing players are at the baseline.

Take It to the Court

WINNING OBJECTIVES

Some of these objectives will likely be modified as you develop into an advanced player, but provide a solid framework for beginning your pickleball journey and will continue to serve you well at all levels of play.

Your objectives in every game are to take the offensive position by getting to the NVZ, staying there unless forced back by a well-hit lob, working with patience to create a fault from the opposition or a set-up for a winning shot, and putting the ball away to win the rally.

1. When serving, aim to serve the ball deep 100 percent of the time, unless you are specifically targeting the short corner.
2. When receiving, return the served ball slow and deep. Immediately after you hit the ball, move forward quickly to the NVZ line so that you're side by side with your partner. An exception to look for is an opponent, usually the server's partner, who moves forward as the serve is struck. Your return has to bounce (the "two-bounce rule") before they hit it, so a harder, deep drive aimed at or past the out-of-position player, between them and the baseline, can be an easy winner. Even if they manage to backpedal and return it, their shot is likely to be a weak one.
3. When on the serving team, wait for the ball to bounce after the serve is returned, then hit an equalizing third shot of the rally—preferably a drop shot—which allows both your team members to move safely and quickly (but not rushing or out of control) to the NVZ line.
4. If and when all four players are established at the net, dinking the ball back and forth, aim your shots to areas that make your opponents' returns more difficult, encouraging them to make an error. Look for and hit aggressively downward the first ball that comes to you high enough. How high is "high enough" is another thing that will change as your game develops. Many beginners need to have a ball well above the net before they have much chance of successfully driving the ball down for a winner. More and more advanced players are using enough topspin to consistently hit a ball hard from below the net tape and still have it dip down into the opposite court with speed and power. This takes practice, with both topspin forehands and backhands.

5. It has become common training language in pickleball to refer to a "high enough" ball—one giving you a likely success in attacking aggressively—as a "green light" ball. "Yellow" balls are less likely to be successfully attacked, so "proceed with caution." "Red lights" are lower shots that must be hit upward to get back over the net. Red lights are perfect opportunities to use tactical, consciously aimed dinks and drops (or perhaps a lob) that can put the opponent at a disadvantage and increase the chance they will commit an error.

MASTERING THE MENTAL GAME

Much has been written about the importance of training the mind as well as the body in preparation for athletic competition. Television and the internet offer a wealth of coverage of both collegiate and professional sports, allowing viewers to see not only the physical abilities of athletes but also the mental and emotional skills that allow them to control themselves in both positive and negative situations. Given two athletes who are equal in ability and knowledge of a sport, the one who is completely focused on the job at hand—choosing and successfully hitting the next shot—as well as completely in control of thoughts and actions will win the game.

As more people have become aware and appreciative of the role of mental training in preparing for sport competition, athletes at all levels have embraced it. Even though most pickleball players are not in training for the next Olympics or world championships, many of those who play the game every day are discovering ways to use mental training to improve their game. Playing as well as you're capable of is nearly always more fun.

Many books are available on the value of mental training. Terry Orlick's 2008 book, *In Pursuit of Excellence*, published by Human Kinetics, belongs at the top of the list. Terry describes the mindset, strategies, and activities of those who are successful in sport and in life this way:

> *Great performers do not begin their lives or pursuits as great performers. They work at getting into a habit of seeing things in positive ways and imagining themselves performing and executing technical skills in the way that they would like to perform them. In fact, most of the best performers in the world have highly developed imagery skills because they use these skills daily to create a positive focus for excel-*

lence. They draw on positive memories, recall the focus and feelings of previous best performances, and create positive visions of the future. They use their positive thoughts and positive imagery to prepare themselves mentally for quality practice, quality performance, and joyful life experiences.

To improve future performances, they carefully revisit positive parts of their current or past performances (so that they know what is working) and assess parts of their performances that can be improved so that they can make necessary adjustments. They often refine or improve their skills by running them through their minds. They think, see, feel, or imagine themselves making the improvement and being competent, confident, successful, and in control, which sets the stage for higher-quality performance. When learning new skills, procedures, routines, or tactics or when making refinements, they often run the desired actions through their minds many times, with quality and feel, to speed up the learning process. Some of them also use positive imagery to relax themselves or regain control when distracted. (p. 17)

The value of mental training in athletic competition is well documented. Hours before you play, maybe even the night before your first tournament game, assume a relaxed position in a comfortable setting. Clear your mind of all the clutter that accumulated during that day. When your body is completely relaxed and your mind is clear, think about the best serve you ever executed. What did it feel like? How did your muscles feel? How were you holding the paddle—with what part of your hand? Where were you looking? Were you feeling especially energetic that day? And then think about your best low, hard drive, your best softly arcing dink landing near a backhand-side foot, that exquisitely angled overhead smash, and so on. How quick were you in getting to the net? Think through every part of your best game. Then tell yourself, "I'm going to duplicate that tomorrow—no problem." Then do it!

Gigi LeMaster uses mental training in her pickleball play in a slightly different way. She focuses on her opponents as well as herself. Gigi won gold medals in women's doubles and mixed doubles in the 2013 Tournament of Champions in Ogden, Utah, in September 2013. Gigi describes her approach this way:

I visualize the shots that I know this particular player has [and] mentally check off how I can answer, neutralize, or counteract those shots.

LeMaster emphasizes the need to let go of mistakes:

After committing an unforced error, I want that shot back, but I move on mentally. I forget about it almost instantly. Mental focus on the shot to come is much more important. I will make a mental note if it's something I can prevent the next time around.

Another player who places a lot of emphasis on the mental side of competition is Jennifer Lucore. A multiple medal winner in 2011, 2012, 2013, and 2014, Jennifer explains the importance of controlling focus:

[Y]our mind must be centered entirely on the match. Ignore anything else that can cause you to get distracted. This includes your opponent's idiosyncrasies—that sometimes requires stronger mental toughness than dealing with your own demons.

The idea of maintaining this level of focus is to keep yourself in the now, in the present, to maximize your performance and stop the interference of mental hurdles. Keep the dialogue between you and your partner strictly focused on what is happening in the game, mainly because that is the only thing you can control at the moment.

As you learn the game of pickleball, you are exposed to a variety of behaviors on the court. There are players whose facial expressions don't change a bit, whether they have just hit a winning shot down the line or sent the ball into the net on the serve. They're happy to win a game but they're also gracious about it. These are the players who focus on the "now" of the game and therefore maintain a classy demeanor on the court, win or lose. Then there are players who can be heard for miles around every time they commit an error. These are often the same players who pat themselves on the back after killing a ball that was set up for them perfectly by the opposition. If they win the match, they tell others about it for weeks; if they lose, it's because of the wind or they just didn't feel well that day. This type of player doesn't realize that getting so upset over making an error bolsters the confidence of opponents. Wes Gabrielsen, gold medalist in the 2013 and 2014 USAPA National Tournaments in 19+ men's singles, 19+ men's doubles, and 19+ mixed doubles, says this:

> *I believe that a player's demeanor on the court is everything. If I see an opponent get frustrated during a match, I know that I have achieved a small victory and that I only need to execute the fundamentals in order to win the match.*

Pickleball, like other sports, places you in a situation where you're forced into reacting to your own successful moves and those of your partner as well as reacting to unsuccessful ones. You, and only you, can decide how you react to those moves and consequently the character you display to others. Keeping winning and losing in proper perspective is a challenge for some of the competitive souls out there, but both experiences are part of the game for everyone. As many have said, pickleball is just a game, and games are supposed to be fun. So get out there and have some fun!

Give It a Go

PRACTICE THE IDEAL DOUBLES SEQUENCE

Practicing the ideal initial three-shot sequence in a controlled situation helps make it automatic for you in a competitive situation. Get together with three other players who, like you, want to learn and practice the sequence. Before the ball is contacted on each serve, focus on your role in that particular rally. What will your next shot be? What should it feel like? Where should you aim? Strengthen or loosen your grip depending on your next anticipated shot. Remind yourself about what you should focus on. Talk to yourself!

- Server: "My first shot is the serve. My second shot, if the ball comes to me, will be a drop shot, or a low, hard drive down the middle, after which I go to the net with my partner."
- Server's partner: "I stay back by the baseline while my partner serves. If the return of the serve comes to me, I return it off the bounce with a drop shot or drive, after which I go to the net with my partner."
- Receiver of serve: "I return the serve slow and deep and then go to the NVZ line to join my partner and get ready for the next shot."
- Receiver's partner: "I'm in a ready position at the NVZ line. I track the ball as it's served and then returned by my partner, looking for an 'out' serve for them so they can concentrate on their return. I'm ready for my first shot, which will be either a volley or a dink."
- And every single player, on every shot, should adopt a balanced ready position, paddle out in front of them and poised for a quick response to any shot coming their way.

S1 serves the ball to R1. R1 returns the serve slow and deep to S2 (figure 10.9) and then moves to the NVZ line.

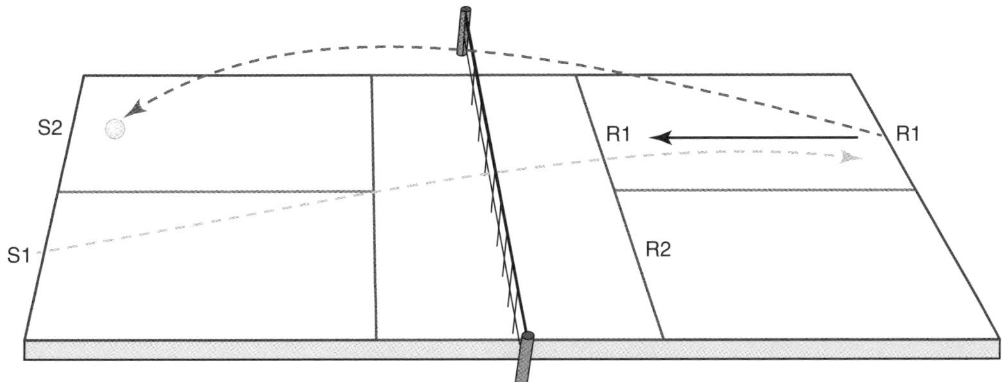

Figure 10.9 Serve and serve return.

S2 hits a drop shot to the middle of the court (figure 10.10), then both S1 and S2 move quickly to the NVZ line.

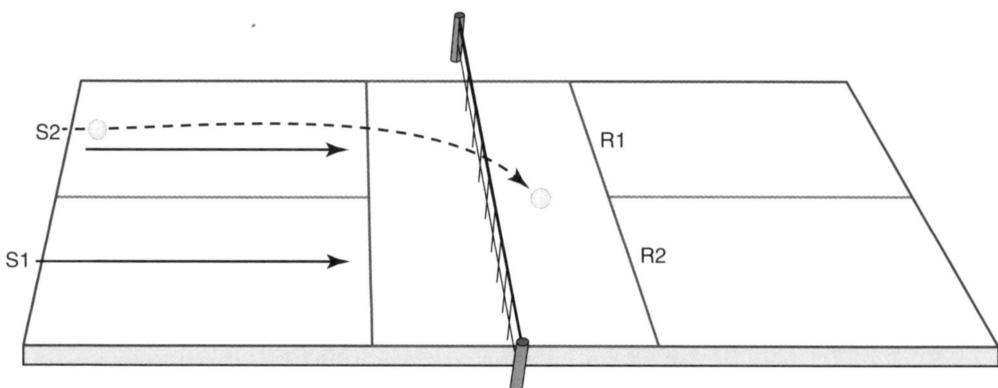

Figure 10.10 Drop shot.

S1, S2, R1, and R2 are all at the net. R2 dinks to S2. S2 dinks to R1 (figure 10.11), who then dinks to S1.

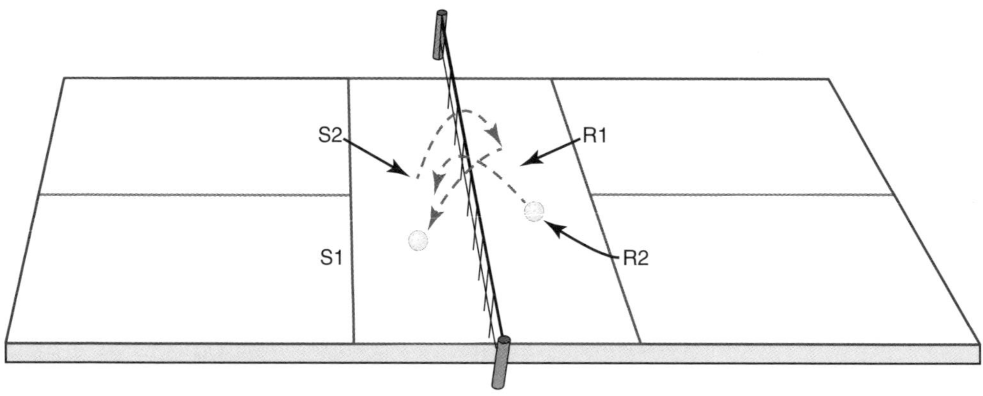

Figure 10.11 Dinking at the net.

S1 dinks crosscourt to R1. R1 hustles over to get it. In an attempt to dink it back, R1 hits the ball too high. S2 sees that it's high, checks to be sure of being outside the NVZ—and volleys it aggressively down the middle of the receiving team's court (figure 10.12). *Point!* (But since this is just a practice, no point!)

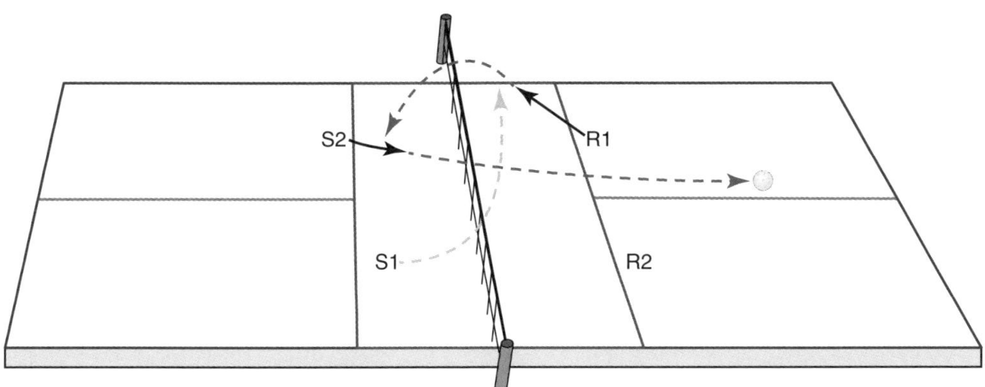

Figure 10.12 Kill shot and point.

Return to your previous serve positions and have the same server serve the ball again. Have that server serve three times to start the shot sequence. Play out each rally, but don't score points. Then have the same server serve three times from the left side. After those six rallies, give the serve to the other side. They then do the same thing. At this point, two of the four players have served. Players on each team switch positions with partners so that the player who hasn't yet served now serves from the right side. Continue this controlled practice until all four players have been in each position.

After you've had an opportunity to practice the ideal shot sequence for doubles and you feel comfortable with it, try it in a game. Having another player complete a checklist (figure 10.13) of the shots you take in the game will help you to evaluate yourself on whether you are using the appropriate shot in a given situation. This frees up your mind so that you can concentrate on the "now"—the current play.

Figure 10.13 Shot Selection Checklist

Name	Serve	Return of serve	Third shot
Key D=Deep MC=Midcourt E=Error	D=Deep MC=Midcourt E=Error	D=Deep MC=Midcourt E=Error	DR=Drop shot GR=Ground-stroke L=Lob E=Error

From USA Pickleball, 2025, *Pickleball Fundamentals, Second Edition* (Champaign, IL: Human Kinetics).

Each checker will watch one or two players. Record in the appropriate column the location of the shot or, in the case of the third shot, the kind of shot taken. The purpose is to evaluate the success of these four players in following a sequence of shots which allows them to get to the NVZ line. Only the first three shots of the rally should be recorded. This is meant to be a controlled practice of the first three shots of a rally—not a game!

Match Point

Playing competitive pickleball by successfully executing the three-shot sequence is a stepping-stone to success and a worthy goal for all players. You may reach that goal many times and you may not, but working consciously toward that goal, honing the effectiveness and consistency of each of those three initial shots, will make you a better player. Be persistent! Simulate the pressures and environment of a tournament game in every practice session. Prepare the same way physically and mentally each time, and eventually you'll discover that your approach to tournament competition is focused, confident, and relaxed.

CHAPTER

11

Strategies for Doubles and Singles Play

As you learn and perfect the skills of pickleball and play more competitive games, you will quickly appreciate how much more there is to it than hitting the ball back and forth across the net. The first time you're successful in placing the ball just over the net when your opponents are deep in their court; or when you pass your opponents with a well-placed down-the-line groundstroke; or when you create an opening in their defense, then place your shot into it for an easy winner—you will feel a tremendous sense of accomplishment and excitement. You were able to do this, and will do it again in the future, because you were persistent in learning new skills and were conscientious about applying the tactics and strategies of the game.

Pickleball players vary in terms of their objectives for playing the game—from the recreational player whose only goal is to get exercise in a fun, social way to the competitive tournament player striving to win a gold medal. There's room for all on the pickleball court. Regardless of what category you're in, though, the process of learning the game and then playing well is the same. You must be able to control the ball coming off your paddle, and you should be able to execute each skill and know when to use it in a game. This is when you reap the benefits of strategic play.

Making plans before a game about hitting to Jane's backhand or dropping the ball short over the net because John tends to not come to the NVZ is of no value if the players in this conversation are erratic and unable to control their play. That's like a catcher in baseball signaling for a curveball to be thrown on the outside corner of the plate when the pitcher has absolutely no control over where any of his pitches go—let alone a curveball! In any game, you must be able to execute the required skills with some degree of consistency before you can hope to use strategy effectively during competition.

You Can Do It

DOUBLES STRATEGIES FROM LEADING PLAYERS.

Following are strategies and comments from Alex Hamner and Jennifer Lucore, 2011, 2012, 2013, and 2014 national women's doubles and singles open champions.

Go for the "W" using these proven hints to improve your doubles game. While some items may come naturally to you, they may not to your partner. So get out there and practice!

Our suggestions are not in any particular order, and we suggest you practice just one or two at a time. If you think too much, pretty soon nothing seems to go right . . . and that's no fun.

- **Move up to and back from the net together, as a team.** *Obviously, when your team is receiving, one of you is already at the kitchen line. So after the serve is returned deep, that person needs to get to the kitchen with her partner. Get moving—points are won when you are at the net together.*
- *But when you are the serving team, wait until the third shot is hit and then both of you, together, move forward and get to the kitchen together. Keep your partner in your peripheral view so you know you are together, because if one of you runs forward and one stays back, you have created a nice hole for your opponents to hit through.*

- **Move left and right together, both at the baseline and at the net.** *Similar to moving up and back together, you need to move left and right together. Again, keep your partner in your peripheral vision. If one of you moves wide and the other stays where they are, you've created a hole for your opponents. For example, if your partner takes three steps to the right to get a wide ball, you may need to take perhaps two steps to fill in the hole that was created. And then you both would move left to prepare for the next shot. Always be on your toes and be ready to do the left or right shuffle.*
- **Don't let anything through the middle.** *This is true regardless of whether you are at the baseline or in the kitchen. You're playing pickleball to hit the ball, right? So go for it! Think "mine," not "yours," when it comes to balls in the middle. It's definitely better for both of you to try to hit the ball than for neither of you to go for it.*
- **Communicate, communicate, communicate**. *It doesn't have to be super loud, but it is super helpful to say things like, "Got it," "Mine," and "I go." But if it's out of your reach, then communicate that, saying, "Yours!" and "You go." If a ball looks like it's going to go out, don't call "out" to your partner. That could lose you a point if it actually lands in. Instead, say things like "Bounce it," "Let it go," or "Watch it." In doubles there should actually be quite a bit of talk on the court. For a ball close to the net that you can't get, say "Get it!" loudly to your partner.*
- **Once you're at the kitchen, stay there**. *If you take a step back to hit a dink that has landed deep, be sure to step back to the kitchen line. If you don't, you may eventually find yourself in no-man's-land! And since you are now moving together as a team, you don't want your partner backing up also. What's so bad about no-man's-land? Virtually never is a point won from that part of the court.*
- **Unforced errors happen!** *Nobody means to hit an unforced error, and nobody likes it. If you make a mistake, own up to it: "Sorry, partner!" And if your partner makes one, support her by being positive: "Good try" or "You'll get it the next time." If you notice why the error was made and think your partner might not be aware of the problem, nicely suggest a correction—maybe your partner is leaning back at contact instead of transferring weight forward, or perhaps instead of bending at the knees, she was bent over at the waist. Or maybe it was just a mistake. Forget it and move on. There's always the next point.*
- **Have fun!** *Pickleball is the best. Enjoy being on the court, swinging away at that plastic ball, being social, and getting exercise all at once. There are definitely worse places you can be than on a pickleball court, so while you are there, get your game on and have fun!*

More to Choose and Use

KEEPING THE BALL IN PLAY

Not enough can be said about the value of keeping the ball in play, a feat that is accomplished by decreasing unforced errors in a game. Consider three statistics cited in *The Official Pickleball Handbook* (1999) by Mark Friedenberg:

1. Three of every four rallies (75 percent) are won or lost because of errors.
2. One of every four rallies (25 percent) are actually earned or won by a good "winner" shot.
3. Three of every four errors (75 percent) are made at the baseline by hitting the ball into the net or out of bounds.

Though these statistics change over the years as tactics vary, the conclusion is the same: keeping the ball in play, forcing your opponents take another shot, giving them another opportunity to make an error, is a winning strategy in pickleball.

Too often, beginning players trying to make the perfect shot attempt to hit the ball too low (and too hard) over the net; not surprisingly, they often fall short of perfection and consequently the ball goes into the net or goes long, past the baseline. The same goes for shots aimed to land on or just inside the boundary lines: it's too easy for the shot to go "out." A far more effective approach is to make keeping the ball in play your main objective, ideally landing near the opponents' feet or in another spot that will make their return more challenging and less aggressive. Even if your return isn't perfect and it ends up being a setup for an aggressive smash from the opponents, you have placed the burden of keeping the ball in play on the opponents and it is possible that their smash could go into the net! It happens more than you might think when a player gets too excited about an "easy" put-away shot suddenly offered to them on a silver platter.

As you're learning the game, use those shots that are considered to be high-percentage shots. Because the net is lower in the middle of the court (34 inches) than it is over the sidelines (36 inches), you should hit the majority of your shots over the middle of the net. This usually means a diagonal path for the ball. The court and the NVZ are both also longer along this diagonal, so shots crossing over the lowest part of the net will also offer more forgiveness if your shot is a little on the long side. As your game improves and your play becomes more consistent, then you can try for more challenging shots.

Take It to the Court

BASIC DOUBLES STRATEGIES

While the best players may use doubles game strategies automatically, they, too, were beginners at one time. Select one or two strategies to work on; when they become automatic to you and your partner, work on one or two more. Eventually your team will truly be one working together toward a common goal: success!

- *Strive for 100 percent accuracy on serves.* The serve is the only shot in the game that is uncontested— the receiving team must let the ball bounce before it can be hit (the first bounce of the two-bounce rule). Therefore, there is no excuse for not serving the ball over the net into the proper court. Your first objective should be to serve with close to 100 percent accuracy. Once you accomplish that, then you can focus on a more aggressive serve and place the shot to your advantage. Don't try to get too fancy with your serve too soon. On the other side, don't beat yourself up if you miss a couple serves. One of the surest ways to make an error is to dwell on a previous error rather than accepting it and making an adjustment as needed going forward.
- *Generally, when both partners are right-handed or both left-handed, the player with the forehand shot has the primary responsibility for balls down the middle.* Even though, as Alex and Jennifer said, it's better for both players to go for the ball rather than neither one trying for it, balls down the middle are the primary responsibility of the player whose forehand is down the middle. This is a guideline and not a rule, and it is more true near the baseline than at the NVZ. Most players' forehands are stronger than backhands, so allowing the player whose forehand is in position to hit the ball can enable your team to return the ball with the strongest possible shot. Experience will show, though, that sometimes the backhand has a better shot at a ball coming over the middle, especially when following a diagonal path. There are several popular and competing theories on how best to determine who should take those middle balls near the net in competitive play, but "forehand takes the middle" is a good summation of the basics that is easy to understand and apply for newer players. This is an important subject to be discussed and agreed upon with any partner you play with regularly. Remember that when one player is left-handed and the other right-handed, both partners will have forehands down the middle or neither will.

- *Anticipate what the return shot will be and move into position to cover the possible angle of the return shot.* With experience, the location of your opponents on the court, their paddle positions and the body position of the player hitting the ball, and the possible angles for the return shot will tell you what the shot will probably be and where it will be hit. Be prepared to move into position for the return early, anticipating the opponent's likely shot. For example, if you and your partner are at the NVZ and one of you has executed a popped-up mishit that will be a setup for a smash, instead of maintaining your position at the net, both of you should move back slightly as time allows, holding paddles at a low, ready, blocking position, with the intention that one of you will be able to get your paddle on the ball, blocking it as it is smashed back across the net, either before or (easier) after it bounces. (figure 11.1).

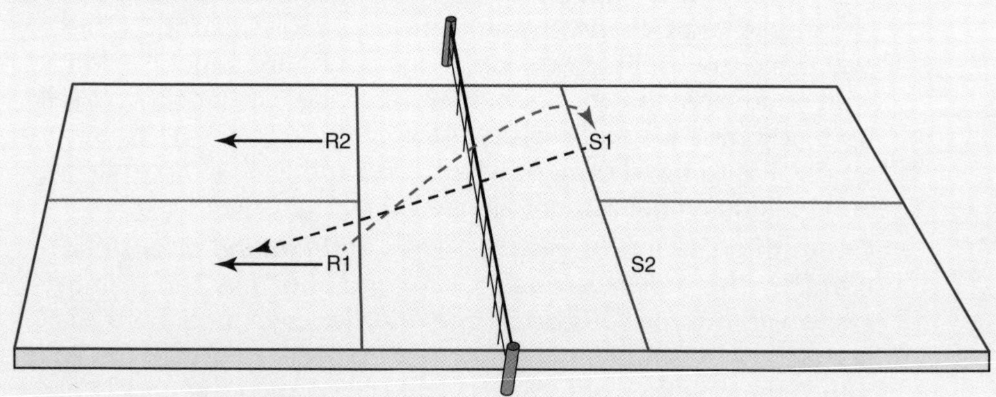

Figure 11.1 Covering the angle of the return.

- *Always face the ball on the other side of the net, with your body and your paddle.* Regardless of where you are on the court and where the ball is on the other side of the net, assume a position that is always facing the ball with the paddle ready, up, out away from your body, and prepared for the ball to be hit to you.
- *Know where you are on the court and where the boundary lines are.* Many beginners will hit any ball coming to them regardless of the flight of the oncoming ball and where they are standing on the court. Every time you hit a ball that would have gone out of bounds, you're extending the rally when, had you let the ball hit the ground first, you would have won the rally. Sometimes, in the heat of an exciting, competitive rally, it can be quite difficult to *not* swing, even if doing nothing, just letting their ball go out, is all that was needed to win.

- *Always strive for placement and control rather than speed when you hit the ball.* The more games that you play, the better you will be able to see where your opponents are on the court. As the ball is coming to you, note where your opponents are and in what direction they're moving (*if* they're moving). Then place the ball at their current location, behind them, or into an open space on their court. If one partner is moving and the other is still and ready, it is almost always a better decision to target the moving player, since they will likely have more difficulty making an effective return with their feet in motion.

ADVANCED DOUBLES STRATEGIES

When you and your partner both feel confident that you're playing a smart game and you're satisfied with your teamwork, you can start thinking about using more advanced strategies, such as poaching, stacking, switching, and hand signals. Don't force their use, as they can be distracting and initially lead to more errors, but when the opportunity to use them arises in recreational or practice games, give them a try.

Poaching

If one partner is already at the net—especially on the left side while facing the net for right-handers—with the other partner still coming to the net but not there yet, and the opposing team is pretty predictable about where their groundstroke is going, the net player can poach by moving across in front of their partner, staying behind the NVZ line and hitting the ball just after it crosses the net (R2 in figure 11.2). The advantage of poaching is that the ball is returned more quickly and more offensively than it would be if it were allowed to continue on to the partner who is still advancing toward the NVZ line. A disadvantage of poaching is

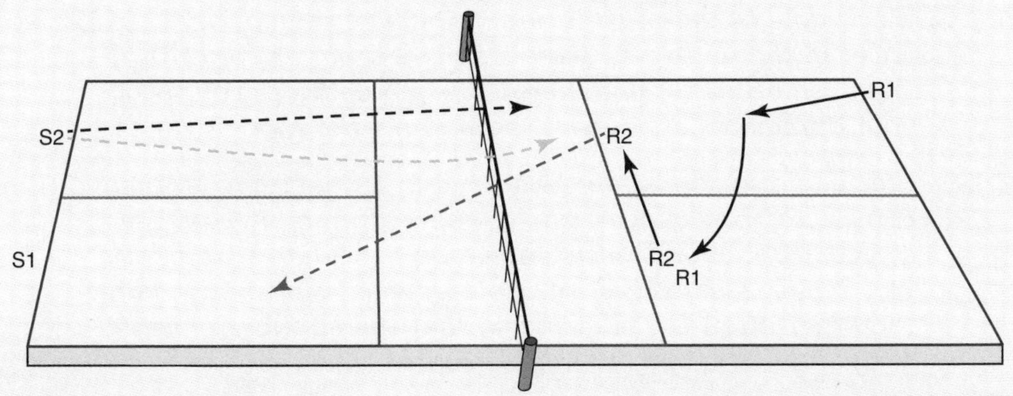

Figure 11.2 Poaching.

that if the opposing team suspects that the net player is going to move across to poach, they may hit a line shot behind the poaching player. Poaching can occur on either side, but is usually a stronger shot if the ball is hit by the forehand of the player poaching.

A common saying holds that "if you poach in front of me, you had better hit a winner." This is not true. Sometimes the poach is the right shot to take and it can give your team an advantage even if it is not an immediate winner. You should be looking for shots that build an advantage for your team, keeping your opponents on the defensive where they are more likely to give you an opening, rather than a more risky attempt to go "from 0 to 60" with a lower-percentage immediate kill shot.

Stacking

Every year, more players of all ages become interested in competing against others in local, regional, national, and international tournaments. In preparation for that competition, players explore ways to improve their chances of winning. One of these is to use stacking. Simply put, stacking means that during the serve, the stronger player, whose forehand should conventionally be down the middle, lines up either at the baseline or at the NVZ line to the left (facing the net) of his partner. If the doubles team consists of one right-handed player and one left-handed player, the right-handed player would always line up to the left of his left-handed partner, keeping both forehands down the middle.

Jim Hackenberg, winner of multiple gold medals in men's doubles and mixed doubles, notes that more pickleball doubles teams are stacking and explains two situations in which it is particularly beneficial:

> *The first relates to a doubles team that consists of a left-handed player and a right-handed player. Stacking allows them to keep both of their forehands down the middle all the time. As most players know, hitting the ball down the middle of the court is one of the best shots. The net is lower in the middle so there's a higher margin for error if you mishit the shot and there is the possibility of confusing your opponents about who should take the shot.*
>
> *Stacking also can be an advantage to a doubles team that consists of one player who is more dominant—quicker, stronger, and more consistent—than the other. Mixed-doubles teams that consist of a player who is stronger than the other often use stacking so that the stronger player's forehand is covering all middle shots.*

The rules pertaining to the serve and the return of the serve apply to the two players involved in the serve and return action, not their partners. So while the server must stand behind the baseline and behind the proper service court, the server's partner can stand anywhere. Similarly, the player receiving the serve should be in a position that will allow for a return of serve, but the receiving player's partner can be anywhere on or just off their court.

Jim considers that there are stacking variations ranging from a full stack, a 75 percent stack, and a serving (defensive) half stack. For a 75 percent stack, your team would stack in all instances except when the weaker player is receiving the serve behind the left service court. If your team chose to use a serving (defensive) stack, you would stack only when your team is serving; with this option, both players would receive serves normally. Stacking requires practice and also more running and exertion than conventional positioning, but it is effective, as its regular use by successful players at all competitive levels attests.

Figure 11.3 illustrates the way players would stack in various situations.

Situation	Position before serve	Action after serve
Stronger player serving from right	Sp Wp	Stronger player slides left
Stronger player serving from left	Sp Wp	Standard
Weaker player serving from right	Sp Wp	Standard
Weaker player serving from left	Sp Wp	Weaker player slides rights
Stronger player receiving from right	Sp Wp	Stronger player runs to non-volley zone line on left
Stronger player receiving from left	Sp Wp	Standard
Weaker player receiving from right	Sp Wp	Standard
Weaker player receiving from left	Sp Wp	Weaker player runs to non-volley zone line on right

Figure 11.3 Stacking chart.

Jim offers this advice to players who are considering stacking:

The advantages of stacking are fairly easy to identify—both players hit more shots with their forehands, and the dominant player has more opportunities to cover a larger area of the court. The disadvantages are also pretty simple to identify—partners forget where they are supposed to be! Nothing is worse than losing a point by being out of position. Never enter a tournament and try to stack if you haven't practiced it several times with your partner. Just as you need to practice the other skills of the game, you also need to practice stacking. Have the first server wear a red wristband just like in a tournament. After a rally, ask yourself what your score is. The answer will tell you which partner is where. Your first server with the wristband will be behind the right service court (facing the net) any time your score is even and behind the left service court when your score is odd. With practice, stacking becomes a valuable tool.

Consider this when playing a team that is stacking: they are likely trying to load their best weapons (almost always forehands) in the middle of the court. They likely do not have as much confidence in their backhands. Stacking means that these potentially weaker shots will always be positioned toward the sidelines. Consider playing more of your shots toward their weakness on the outside rather than repeatedly feeding their loaded middle forehands. In other words: don't give them the shot they want. Instead, take advantage of their weaker areas and their unwittingly broadcasting where these weaknesses may be.

Putting Spin on the Ball

Once your pickleball game becomes consistent and you feel confident that you can control the speed and direction of the ball coming off your paddle, you will likely want to experiment with putting more spin on the ball. A topspin or a backspin on groundstrokes, a sidespin on a serve, and a backspin on dinks can all be very effective. Advanced players often hit the return of serve with a slicing combination of sidespin and backspin that can make the third shot tougher to execute. (See the More to Choose and Use section in chapter 3 for details on applying spin.)

Give It a Go

SINGLES STRATEGIES

The obvious difference between playing pickleball doubles and singles is that a singles game involves only one player competing against another. The game still consists of one player scoring 11 points and being at least 2 points ahead of the opponent, and a match is the best 2 out of 3 games. When the server's score is even, the serve is from behind the right service court (as the server faces the net); when the score is odd, the server serves from behind the left service court. The skills are the same, although in singles soft shots at the net are not as prevalent as in doubles. The server stands right next to the center line in order to easily move either to the right or left to get to the return shot.

Because there are long rallies of dinking in doubles but not in singles, a competitive pickleball match in doubles takes about twice as long as a match in singles. Playing pickleball singles successfully requires a player not only to be in good physical condition but also to be able to anticipate the next shot from the opponent. There is no partner to help cover the court, so if the competing player can get a jump on moving in the correct direction of the next shot, it's definitely to the player's advantage. Most players start out playing doubles and then move on to singles if they are interested in a more challenging experience. Singles is more similar to tennis, with players tending to stay closer to the baseline and often driving the ball low and harder than in doubles play.

In 2013, in his first year of competition in the USAP national tournament, Wes Gabrielsen won several gold medals in men's singles, men's doubles, and mixed doubles. Wes highlights the following strategies as keys to singles play:

- *Change the direction and speed of the ball as much as possible.* You want to keep your opponent off balance and running as much as you can. Use a mixture of spins, slices, depth, and angles.
- *Take advantage of your opponent's weaknesses.* If you know that your opponent has a weak backhand or is hesitant to move quickly in a certain direction, exploit that weakness. Always use your strengths against the opponent's weaknesses.
- *Be aggressive.* Follow up a return of the serve by going to the NVZ line. By being at the net, you are decreasing the target area your opponent could hit to and putting pressure on your opponent to hit a passing shot. If you have an opening for a put-away shot, take it!

- *Hit your serves and groundstrokes deep.* A deep, hard-driven serve or groundstroke keeps your opponent deep in his court. You want to keep the opponent away from the net and prevent the player from assuming an offensive position.
- *Play your game.* Make sure that you stick to your game plan and don't let yourself play the kind of game that is the strength of your opponent. Stay in control with a confident mindset.

Wes notes that anyone aspiring to play singles must be in good physical condition. He suggests playing a lot of singles before entering a tournament. Three of Wes's favorite drills for singles follow.

FIGURE EIGHT

Player 1 (P1) is on one end of the court and player 2 (P2) is on the other. Player 1 hits all line shots and player 2 hits all crosscourt shots (figure 11.4). Players switch the kind of shot they're hitting. This drill is excellent for ball control and conditioning.

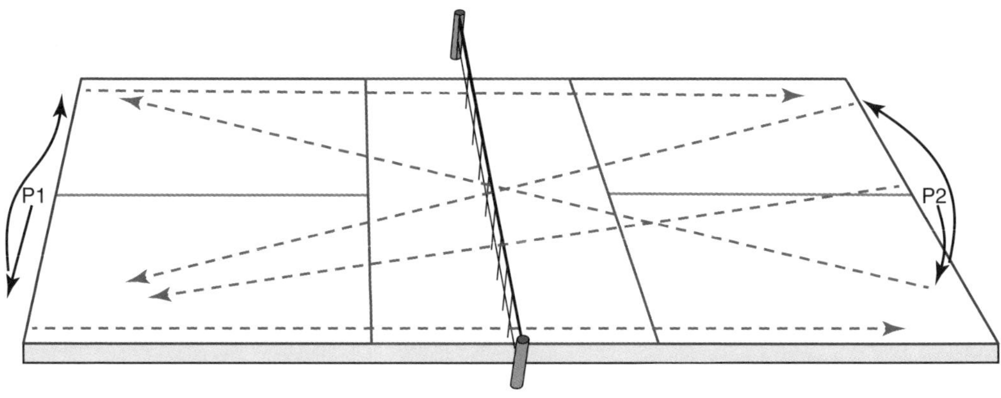

Figure 11.4 Figure eight drill.

FIGURE EIGHT AT THE NET

This is identical to the figure eight except it's played in the kitchen or the NVZ. Player 1 (P1) hits dinks straight across the net and player 2 (P2) hits crosscourt dinks. They then switch the kind of shot they hit (figure 11.5). It's a good drill for conditioning and practicing short, quick moves.

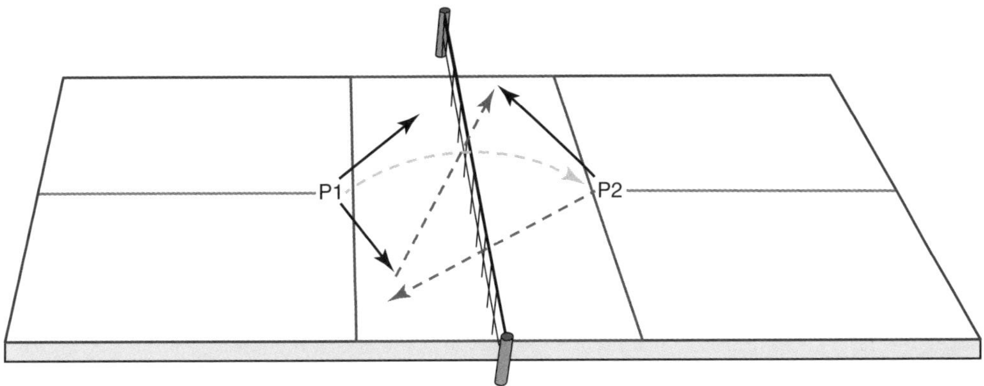

Figure 11.5 Figure eight at the net drill.

WINDSHIELD WIPER

Player 1 (P1) has a basket or ball hopper filled with balls. Player 2 (P2) is at the opposite baseline. P1 feeds balls to P2 and P2 returns each one with a forehand groundstroke and then a backhand groundstroke (figure 11.6). When the basket is empty, they switch positions.

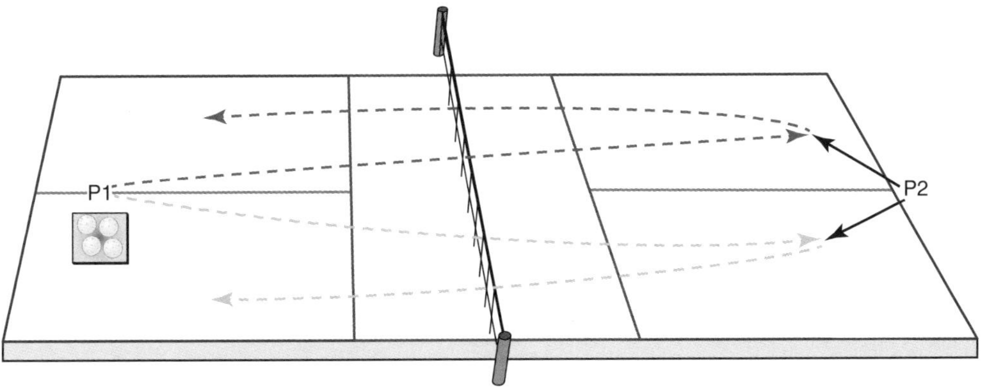

Figure 11.6 Windshield wiper drill.

Match Point

Some players quickly figure out the strategies of the game and are able to use them at the appropriate time. To the majority of players, though, strategies, just like skills, have to be learned and practiced. The most effective way to learn and practice is to watch skilled, experienced players compete against others of equal ability. Videos of recent gold-medal matches in USAP tournaments are available from the USAP website. The USAP has made great strides in producing professionally done videos. YouTube has also exploded in recent years with a wealth of free, informative videos on pickleball matches, drills, and instruction.

Every year more and more pickleball tournaments are held. While tournaments historically grouped competitors by age—19 and older, 35 and older, 50 to 54, 55 to 59, and so on, all the way to 80 and older—almost all tournaments now use a skill rating system in addition to age. The larger tournaments include both age group and skill divisions. Players are rated according to their results against other players in tournaments or any other event that reports results to the various rating agencies. The skill rating system for amateurs is 5.0 (best players), 4.5, 4.0, 3.5, 3.0, and occasionally 2.5 for the newest of competitive players. Most tournaments won't go lower than a 3.0 skill division, and some go no lower than 3.5.

Players competing in their first USAP tournament select the skill level they wish to enter (called "self rating"). It is a good idea to ask a more experienced player who knows your game for advice on this. Competition is held in mixed doubles, men's doubles, and women's doubles; some tournaments offer competition in men's and women's singles. The larger tournaments also offer competition in open divisions, which any player can enter. These tournaments often establish a requirement of minimum skill rating. For example, an open division for men's doubles might include a team of 30-year-olds playing against a team of 70-year-olds, though all players might be required to be at least 4.0 to enter. The open divisions, predictably, are usually the largest in the tournament in terms of the number of entries.

Attending a tournament is the best way to get a feel for what good competitive pickleball is all about. If you can't make it to a tournament, watch the videos, or any challenge court or league games between two of your top local teams. Regardless of whether you're there in person or watching the play on your computer, focus on why the good teams are winning. Then, when you go back to your own courts to play, focus on only one or two strategies every time you play. One day it can be communicating with your partner. The next time, work on getting to the net quickly and side by side with your partner. Eventually those tactics will become automatic. As that happens, you will see much improvement in your overall game.

If you want more action and are eager to pit your playing ability against the ability of a lone competitor, give singles play a try. Being able to play both pickleball singles and doubles with success is an admirable accomplishment.

ABOUT USA PICKLEBALL

USA Pickleball is the national governing body for the sport of pickleball in the United States and provides players with official rules, tournaments, rankings, and promotional materials. Its mission is to promote the development and growth of pickleball in the United States and its territories.

The association is a nonprofit 501(c)(3) corporation and is governed by a board of directors and professional staff who provide guidance and infrastructure for the continued growth and development of the sport.

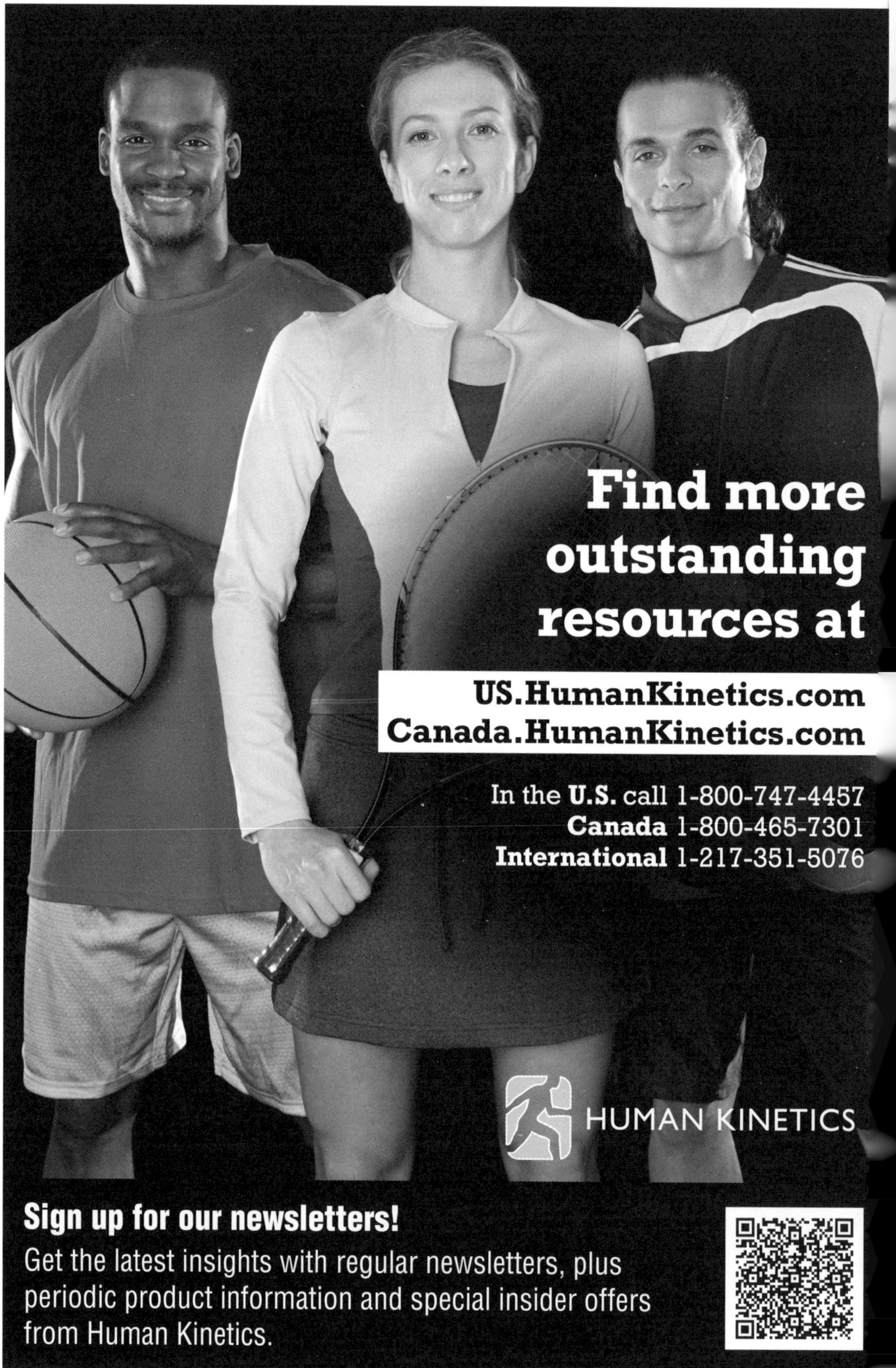

PICKLEBALL FUNDAMENTALS

SECOND EDITION